Parisa M. Garrett
Kahyun Yoon-Flannery

Editors

A Pediatrician's Path

What to Expect After a Pediatrics Residency

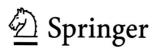 Springer

Editors
Parisa M. Garrett
Philadelphia Department
of Public Health
Ambulatory Health Services
Philadelphia, PA
USA

Kahyun Yoon-Flannery
Janet Knowles Breast
Cancer Center
MD Anderson Cancer Center at
Cooper
Camden, NJ
USA

ISBN 978-3-030-75369-6   ISBN 978-3-030-75370-2 (eBook)
https://doi.org/10.1007/978-3-030-75370-2

This Springer imprint is published by the registered company Springer Nature
Switzerland AG
The registered company address is: Gewerbestrasse 11, 6330 Cham, Switzerland

For Mike, Ellie, and Audrey

For Peter, Ella, Leo, Max, and Nathan

And for all the healthcare workers fighting both in the frontlines and behind the scenes of the COVID-19 pandemic

Preface

This book came together in 2020, amid a global pandemic. Our lives were changed as cities experienced lockdowns, children transitioned to virtual school, many lost their jobs, and the political divide widened. Yet through it all, physicians continued working without a second thought. We showed up for our patients despite fear of bringing the disease home to our families, despite the trauma of the death toll, through protests, inconsistent leadership, and the spread of misinformation.

This dedication is what you, too, will bring to the field of pediatrics, along with all the clinical knowledge you have accrued along the way. This book is designed to fill in the gaps – to help you navigate the day-to-day details and challenges that are not covered during clinical training. As you will see in the pages that follow, there are many exciting opportunities that await you in your journey as a pediatrician. Our hope is that this book will be a valuable resource for you, not just now as you are completing residency, but as you continue to navigate your career in pediatrics.

Many thanks to our senior editor, Dr. Kay Yoon-Flannery, without whom this book would not exist. When she approached me with the idea for this project, I was excited but did not know what to expect. With time and her guidance, support, and determination, *A Pediatrician's Path* came to fruition.

Thank you also to our authors, many of whom fought on the frontlines of the COVID-19 pandemic while developing their chapter content. 2020 was not an easy year to be a physician, and our authors went above and beyond with their contributions to this book. We are so appreciative of your patience and commitment to this project.

I am grateful for my children, Ellie and Audrey, who helped keep things light during the pandemic. They supported *A Pediatrician's Path* by patiently giving me the time I needed to work on the book, and by agreeing to have their photos included. Most importantly, I want to thank my incredible husband, Mike, who has been my partner and ultimate supporter both in my career and through the ups and downs of life.

Philadelphia, PA, USA   Parisa M. Garrett, MD, FAAP
February 2, 2021

Acknowledgments

This book is the second in our *path* series, providing wisdom from the past experiences of those who stood before us in various fields of medicine. When Dr. Garrett and I first met to discuss this project for budding pediatricians, there were many pages of notes taken, with a flurry of ideas and drafts drawn up. Never did either of us think we would be embarking on this project during a pandemic. But thanks to our dedicated authors' efforts, all the while battling the true enemy that was this pandemic, we were able to meet our deadline with this beautiful book among us.

It would be wrong of me to take any of the credit for the *path* series. My own mentor, Dr. Marc Neff, who fueled my fire for the *Surgeon's Path,* is the reason this series and I are where we are.

Life in medicine, with or without a pandemic, is not an easy road. Whether you are a pediatrician or a surgeon, we make so many sacrifices to be where we are, dedicating our lives to save patients every day. Mistakes can be made – our hope is that perhaps our past experiences can guide new budding pediatricians from repeating the same mistakes we have made.

Lastly, I would like to dedicate this to my family, particularly my eldest child, my daughter Aurelia. She not only conquered the year of juggling between virtual/hybrid/pandemic learning, she really helped manage our crazy household with 3 younger brothers at her tender age of 10. I was always brought up to speak my mind, but my daughter certainly takes it to a new level of speaking her own mind. I am ever more thankful that I am raising such an independent, sassy, outspoken but kind young woman as my daughter.

February 3, 2021   Kahyun Yoon-Flannery, DO, MPH

Contents

Contributors

Dominic Adams, MHA, CPHRM Children's Hospitals of Philadelphia, Philadelphia, PA, USA

Gabriela Andrade, MD The Children's Hospital of Philadelphia, Philadelphia, PA, USA

Jodi Brady-Olympia, MD Division of Adolescent Medicine, Department of Pediatrics, Penn State Children's Hospital, Hershey, PA, USA

Department of Pediatrics, Penn State Children's Hospital, Hershey, PA, USA

Nadia Rao Day, MD Pediatric Associates, PC, Phoenix, AZ, USA

Dmitry Dukhovny, MD, MPH Oregon Health and Science University, Portland, OR, USA

Issy C. Esangbedo, MD, MPH South Philadelphia Health and Literacy Center, Philadelphia, PA, USA

Eileen M. Everly, MD General Pediatrics, The Children's Hospital of Philadelphia, Philadelphia, PA, USA

Parisa M. Garrett, MD, FAAP Philadelphia Department of Public Health, Ambulatory Health Services,, Philadelphia, PA, USA

Mary Glas Gaspers, MD, MPH University of Arizona, Tucson, AZ, USA

Adam Glasofer, MD, MSHI Information Technology, Virtua Health, Marlton, NJ, USA

Kanika Gupta, MD Division of General Pediatrics, Nemours Alfred I. duPont Hospital for Children, Wilmington, DE, USA

Kamilah Halmon, MD Inova Children's Hospital, Falls Church, VA, USA

S. Amna Husain, MD Pure Direct Pediatrics, Marlboro, NJ, USA

Jaime Jump, DO, FAAP Baylor College of Medicine, Houston, TX, USA

Sections of Critical Care and Palliative Care, Texas Children's Hospital, Houston, TX, USA

Erin Teresa Kelly, MD, FAAP, FACP Ambulatory Health Services, Philadelphia Department of Public Health, Philadelphia, PA, USA

Shareen F. Kelly, MD Drexel University College of Medicine, Section of General Pediatrics at St. Christopher's Hospital for Children, Philadelphia, PA, USA

Sarah Kramer, MD Watchung Pediatrics, Warren, NJ, USA

Alla Kushnir, MD Department of Pediatrics, Cooper Children's Regional Hospital, Camden, NJ, USA

Ana Mann, MD Advocare Pediatric Urgent Care, Cherry Hill, NJ, USA

Elizabeth C Maxwell, MD Assistant Professor of Clinical Pediatrics, Perelman School of Medicine, University of Pennsylvania, Philadelphia, PA, USA

Lauren A. McNickle, MD Department of Emergency Medicine, Baystate Medical Center, Springfield, MA, USA

Angela Michaels, MD Department of Pediatrics, Division of Neonatal-Perinatal Medicine, Wake Forest Baptist Health, Winston-Salem, NC, USA

Ellen C. Miele, MD, FAAP Spring Lake Pediatrics, Spring Lake, NJ, USA

Ursula S. Nawab, MD Perelman School of Medicine, Children's Hospital of Philadelphia, Philadelphia, PA, USA

Namrita Odackal, DO Neonatology, North Denver Envision Group, Louisville, CO, USA

Robert P. Olympia, MD Department of Emergency Medicine & Pediatrics, Penn State Hershey Medical Center, Hershey, PA, USA

Jodi Brady Olympia, MD Division of Adolescent Medicine, Department of Pediatrics, Penn State Children's Hospital, Hershey, PA, USA

Department of Pediatrics, Penn State Children's Hospital, Hershey, PA, USA

Andrew Palladino, MD Pfizer, Inc., Collegeville, PA, USA

Shweta Parmekar, MD Baylor College of Medicine, Huston, TX, USA

Stephanie Pearson, MD, FACOG PearsonRavitz, LLC, Ardmore, PA, USA

Krupa Playforth, MD The Pediatrician Mom, Mclean, VA, USA

Amol Purandare, MD, FAAP Pediatric Infectious Diseases, Children's Mercy Hospital, Kansas City, MO, USA

Sharla Rent, MD Duke University, Durham, NC, USA

Kristine Schmitz, MD Department of Pediatrics, St. Christopher's Hospital for Children/Drexel University School of Medicine, Philadelphia, PA, USA

Jennifer Shook, MD Division of Adolescent Medicine, Department of Pediatrics, Penn State Children's Hospital, Hershey, PA, USA

Tanushree Singhal, MD Department of Pediatrics, Mayo Clinic Health System, EAU CLAIRE, WI, USA

Nicole Streeks-Wooden, MD, FAAP Pediatrics, CAMCare Health Corporation, Camden, NJ, USA

Kristin Struble, MD Camelback Pediatrics, PC, Phoenix, AZ, USA

Sarah M. Taub, MD Children's Hospital of Philadelphia, Care Network Norristown, Norristown, PA, USA

Joannie Yeh, MD Sidney Kimmel Medical College, Philadelphia, PA, USA

Kahyun Yoon-Flannery, DO, MPH, FACS Janet Knowles Breast Cancer Center, MD Anderson Cancer Center at Cooper, Camden, NJ, USA

Part I

Pediatric Fellowships

Parisa M. Garrett

Congratulations on nearing completion of your pediatric residency! Are you considering pursuing a subspecialty fellowship? In the following chapters, you will find an overview of the fellowship application process, as well as an introduction to several different fellowship types available to graduates of a pediatric residency. While this is not a comprehensive list, it aims to give a sample of the fellowship experience for those who are considering this path.

Applying for Fellowship

Alla Kushnir

Introduction

You have completed your first year of residency and are now thinking about what the next phase of your career will look like. If you have decided that general pediatrics practice is not for you, what should you do now? The thought of applying again may seem overwhelming, especially when it feels like you have just finished the application process for residency. But fellowship applications and interviews are somewhat different from the residency application process. There are a number of similarities, such as the need to go through ERAS [1] again, fill out a similar application, and request letters of recommendations. However, the main difference is that you are not competing with as many people for one spot, and this process is more like applying for a job than applying for medical school or residency. You have *much* more control.

Decision

How do you know if this is the right move for you? Whatever you choose as your specialty or subspecialty, you will likely practice it for the next 30+ years, so make sure you truly enjoy the field

A. Kushnir (✉)
Department of Pediatrics, Cooper Children's Regional Hospital,
Camden, NJ, USA

© The Author(s), under exclusive license to Springer Nature   3
Switzerland AG 2021
P. M. Garrett, K. Yoon-Flannery (eds.), *A Pediatrician's Path*,
https://doi.org/10.1007/978-3-030-75370-2_1

that you are choosing. Don't settle, and don't rule something out just because the specialty is considered "hard" or "impossible for life-work balance." If you care about life-work balance, and I really hope you do, and you care about the field you choose, you can make any specialty work. Regardless of whether you are considering neonatology, pediatric critical care, hematology/oncology, or any of the other amazing possibilities, you can make it perfect for you. Read on to learn more about specific fields later in this book.

Make sure you speak to a number of physicians in the field, both recent graduates and more senior faculty, to learn the different perspectives. Also, try to do a rotation outside of your hospital in the field of your consideration and in a hospital that is different than yours. If your residency is in a community or rural hospital, do a rotation in an inner city or an urban hospital, and vice versa. This will show you different aspects of the specialty and may be helpful in deciding if it's the right specialty for you.

Try to find someone in the field that you trust and with whom you can be candid. Having a mentor is always important, and it can make your life much easier if you have a senior member of the faculty in your corner.

Application for Fellowship

Now that you have decided on a specific fellowship, what's the next step? See Table 1.1 for the general timeline. The dates are not exact, so use the links below to verify timelines for a particular specialty.

The following pediatric specialties are included in the match [2, 3]:

1. *Academic General Pediatrics (AGP)* (http://www.pedsubs. org/SubDes/AcademicGeneralist.cfm) and (http://academic-peds.org/education/education_fellowships.cfm)
2. *Child Abuse* (www.helfersociety.org)
3. *Developmental-Behavioral Pediatrics* (www.sdbp.org/)

Table 1.1 Timeline for fellowship applications

Date	Activity
Early June	ERAS season begins
Early June	MyERAS tokens are generated and distributed Applicants can register in MyERAS and begin working on their applications
Early July	Fellowship applicants may begin submitting applications
Mid-August to October	Programs may begin interviewing applicants
September	Match opens
End of October	Ranking opens
Late November–early December	Rank order list deadline
Early December	Match day
End of May	ERAS season ends

4. *Neonatal-Perinatal Medicine* (Section on Neonatal Perinatal Medicine and the Organization of Neonatal-Perinatal Medicine Training Program Directors) both of the American Academy of Pediatrics
5. *Pediatric Cardiology* (www2.aap.org/sections/cardiology/default.cfm)
6. *Pediatric Critical Care* (www.pedsccm.org)
7. *Pediatric Emergency Medicine* (http://www2.aap.org/sections/pem/default.cfm)
8. *Pediatric Endocrinology* (www.pedsendo.org/home/)
9. *Pediatric Gastroenterology* (www.naspghan.org)
10. *Pediatric Hematology/Oncology* (www.aspho.org)
11. *Pediatric Hospital Medicine* (http://phmfellows.org/
12. *Pediatric Infectious Diseases* (www.pids.org)
13. *Pediatric Nephrology* (www.aspneph.org)
14. *Pediatric Pulmonology* (http://www2.aap.org/sections/pulmonology/default.cfm)
15. *Pediatric Rheumatology* (http://www2.aap.org/sections/rheumatology/)
16. *Pediatric Transplant Hepatology* (https://www.tts.org/split/split-home)

Table 1.2 Commonly required documents for fellowship applications

ERAS application
Medical school transcript and dean's letter
Minimum of three letters of recommendation, including one letter from residency program director and one of the letters from faculty in the specific field
Personal statement including a description of special interests and career goals
Wallet-size color photograph
USMLE transcripts (Steps 1 & 2 are required; Step 3 is strongly encouraged) or COMLEX transcripts
ECFMG status report (only for International Medical Graduates)
Curriculum vitae (if you don't have one, you should work on it now)

All pediatric fellowships are 3 years in length, except Academic General Pediatrics, Pediatric Emergency Medicine, and Pediatric Hospital Medicine, which are 2 to 3 years. Pediatric Transplant Hepatology is 1 year, but you must first complete a fellowship in Pediatric Gastroenterology after a residency in Pediatrics or Medicine/Pediatrics (Table 1.2).

Interviews

Once all the ERAS documents are submitted and ERAS opens, fellowship programs will begin to evaluate applications. Some programs will invite candidates for interviews on a rolling basis: first come, first invited. Others may wait for a certain number of applications to be evaluated prior to inviting the first set of residents to visit. Unlike in residency, there are not as many choices for interview days, and the interviews last from October to approximately mid- to late November.

Interview day itself is much longer than for residency interviews. It usually starts early in the morning, includes a lunch with the current fellows, and finishes late in the afternoon. Rarely, there is an opportunity for dinner the night before or the night of the interview, but this is not the norm. You are likely to meet many of the faculty with whom you will be closely working, advanced practice providers who are involved in fellow education, as well as other fellows. Please remember that lunch with the fellows is still part of the interview day, and thus you are being "judged" just like the rest of the interview day. That does not mean that you should not take the opportunity to talk to the fellows to get a better sense of what the program is truly like. Remember, you are looking for the perfect fit as much as the program is trying to find a candidate who is a good fit for them.

Because fellowship is much more specialized, the conversation is likely to be more focused. For many programs there is an expectation that you have either done some research or have interest in doing research or quality improvement. You don't need to have done research in your field, but you *must* be able to talk about your research intelligently. It is not enough to recite the title and the aim, you need to be able to discuss it in detail. If you have not had an opportunity to participate in a research project, be ready to discuss why and speak about some specific topics that interest you and that you may be interested in studying (this is not written in stone, so don't stress too much about the specific topic).

Research the physicians that you are likely to interview with. You should know their interests and make sure you at least understand the basic concept behind their work. Learning about the program and the members of the team prior to the interview is not a "gunner" move; it is expected. You should always try to learn about the job where you are planning to spend the next 3 years of your life, especially if you are hoping to learn from the program and the faculty. Make sure the fellowship is a good match for you.

Match

Speaking of a good match, by late November or early December, you will finally be finished interviewing. You may have chosen to interview with each program that granted you an interview because you are applying for a competitive fellowship or you are worried about getting in for other reasons (Visa, grades, lack of experience, etc.). Conversely, you may have been limited by location or other factors and interviewed at only one or two fellowship programs. Now it is time to rank the programs and submit to the match.

Hopefully, you have been keeping track of the most important and distinguishing characteristics of every program. Most are similar, but there are always differences. Are you in one hospital only, or are you responsible for covering two to four different hospitals? Is the location in a city or close to one, or more suburban/rural? Will you be the only fellow for the year or one of many? Is the program completely dependent on the fellows for clinical coverage, and will you be expected to fill in the role of a resident? These, and many others, are all important questions to deliberate when finalizing your rank list. When deciding whether to rank a program or not, consider two situations. Would you rather do a year or two of general pediatrics as you are reapplying or do a fellowship in that particular program? If you are unhappy for 3 years, you will not learn as much as you otherwise would, and those around you will be able to sense your misery.

Remember, you want to reach for what you consider the best option, but also be realistic about your chances. Identify what you may be interested in doing after fellowship, and make your choices with this in mind. For example, if you never want to do basic research, then a program that insists on significant basic research and NIH grants may not be the best first choice. Once you have finalized your rank list, submit it, and good luck!

References

1. Applying to Residencies with ERAS® (aamc.org).
2. ERAS 2021 Participating Specialties & Programs (aamc.org)
3. Fellowship Training (aap.org)

Adolescent Medicine Fellowship

Jodi Brady-Olympia and Jennifer Shook

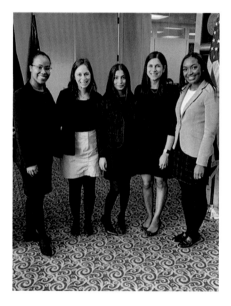

J. Brady-Olympia (✉) · J. Shook
Division of Adolescent Medicine, Department of Pediatrics, Penn State
Children's Hospital, Hershey, PA, USA
e-mail: jbradyolympia@pennstatehealth.psu.edu; jshook1@
pennstatehealth.psu.edu

© The Author(s), under exclusive license to Springer Nature
Switzerland AG 2021
P. M. Garrett, K. Yoon-Flannery (eds.), *A Pediatrician's Path*,
https://doi.org/10.1007/978-3-030-75370-2_2

What Is Adolescence?

Age 10 years to early 20s is commonly referred to as "adolescence." It is not a strictly defined period, but rather a gradual transition from childhood into adulthood. Over this transition, we expect maturation not only physically but also socially and emotionally [1]. At the start of this transition period, we have young children, often concrete in their thinking and heavily dependent on the adults in their lives. At the conclusion of the transition, we expect to have a self-sufficient young adult, able to think and reason abstractly and independently. It is the goal of those caring for adolescents to help facilitate this process and help our patients to navigate this journey successfully.

The History of Adolescent Medicine

The beginnings of comprehensive healthcare for adolescents in the United States can be traced back to the time period just following World War II. Around that time universities began to consider what their role was in providing healthcare for their students [2]. During this period of time, there also arose an interest in studying the normal growth and development as well as mental health of adolescents. In 1941, the American Academy of Pediatrics held a symposium on adolescents during which some of these studies were presented [3]. In the years that followed, the field of Pediatrics, with some contribution from Internal Medicine, began to take on responsibility for improving healthcare available to adolescents [3]. In 1951, Dr. James Roswell Gallagher started the first subspecialty service dedicated to the care of adolescents [2]. In 1952, an Adolescent Unit was launched at the Children's Hospital in Boston, which was a significant development as it highlighted the importance of healthcare dedicated to adolescents [3].

The Society for Adolescent Health and Medicine (SAHM) was founded in 1967 [4]. It was born out of a series of seminars held at the Children's Hospital in Washington, D.C., where the goal was to educate physicians caring for adolescents [3]. Even from the beginning, the importance of multidisciplinary care was recognized with teams of providers including psychologists, nutritionists, social workers, and nurses, in addition to other disciplines [2]. This recognition of the importance of multidisciplinary collaborations in the field of adolescent medicine is apparent even today. The Leaders in Adolescent Health (LEAH) program is a multidisciplinary training program with the goal of mentoring and developing leaders in adolescent health [5]. Funding of the LEAH program by the US Department of Health and Human Services Maternal and Child Health Bureau began in 1977 [5].

Adolescent medicine is recognized as a subspecialty by the American Board of Pediatrics, American Board of Internal Medicine, and the American Board of Family Medicine. The first certifying exam was administered jointly by the American Board of Pediatrics and the American Board of Internal Medicine in 1994 [6]. Both the American Board of Internal Medicine and American Board of Family Medicine require a 2-year training program. The American Board of Pediatrics requires fellows to complete a 3-year program which entails additional time for scholarly activity [7]. The Society for Adolescent Health and Medicine lists 30 adolescent medicine fellowship training programs beginning training in July 2021 (www.Adolescenthealth.org).

What Makes the Subspeciality of Adolescent Medicine Unique from General Pediatrics?

While most general pediatricians care for adolescents in their practice, adolescent medicine specialists receive additional training and experience in areas such as adolescent gynecology, eating disorders, substance use, gender diverse care, and mood disorders. They also often work as part of a multidisciplinary team in caring for adolescents with complex psychosocial concerns in addition to complex medical challenges. In addition, many adolescent medicine specialists practice in academic settings where they are also involved in research and education of medical students, residents, and fellowship trainees.

What Skills or Qualities Are Necessary to Work with Adolescents?

In order to establish rapport with adolescents and effectively communicate with them, there are several skills that are essential. One must understand the transition that takes place in the journey from childhood into adulthood and the developmental steps along that path; thus, a sound knowledge of normal growth and development is crucial. We need to understand how the adolescent is growing and changing through this transitional period both to effectively communicate with them and recognize concerning deviations from what is expected. It is necessary to show the adolescent respect and acknowledge their increasing autonomy as they are entrusted with the responsibility of caring for their own health and overall well-being. On the other hand, it is also important to involve the adolescent's family or other personal or professional supports in their lives. In addition, it is crucial to effectively establish rapport, gaining the adolescent's trust in a professional, nonjudgmental manner. While adolescents may give us answers to our questions, they will be unlikely to discuss deeper concerns, questions, and fears if they do not feel they can trust their healthcare provider. While we are working to gain their trust and establish rapport, it is also important to discuss confidentiality and its limitations as well as make sure that appropriate boundaries are set at the onset of the encounter. This will help create a safe environment for both the adolescent and the provider [1].

Establishing rapport and developing trust are particularly important when working with adolescents when we consider the leading causes of morbidity and mortality. Unintentional injuries, suicide, and homicide continue to be the leading causes of mortality in this age group, and behavioral, social, and environmental factors contribute largely to these leading causes of morbidity and mortality [2]. As a result, the importance of creating a safe environment where they can honestly share their emotions and risk-taking behaviors cannot be overstated. In order to guide them and know what resources they need, it is crucial to understand their emotions and behaviors.

Why Choose a Career in Adolescent Medicine? The Opportunities Are Vast

1. **Adolescent medicine physicians play an important role in guiding their patients as they transition from childhood into adulthood.** They work with other healthcare providers to educate adolescents to take an active role in their own healthcare. As they leave the childhood period where they relied on their parents to make medical decisions, it is our role to partner with them as they learn to ask questions and take on responsibility to make their own medical decisions. With this, it is also important that they gain the skills necessary to advocate for themselves and their needs. They need to learn how the decisions they are making both in the office setting and in their lives can impact their present and future health.

2. **Adolescent medicine physicians are able to counsel and provide guidance and accurate information about many sensitive or high-risk topics.** As they build rapport with the adolescents, adolescents learn that their medical provider is a trustworthy source of accurate medical information and resources in the community.

3. **Adolescent medicine physicians enjoy the challenge of providing medical care to adolescents with complex medical and psychosocial needs.**

4. **Adolescent medicine physicians work as part of an interdisciplinary team.**

5. **Adolescent medicine physicians may work in school-based health clinics.** These clinics can be found in a variety of settings such as colleges or universities, boarding schools, or inner-city schools. In this setting, adolescent medicine physicians may also be involved in sports medicine clinics or act as a team physician.

6. **There are numerous opportunities to participate in research to advance the field of adolescent healthcare both in the United States and around the world.**

7. **There are numerous opportunities to participate in global medicine**. Adolescents make up a large percentage of the population around the world and play a key role in the political,

social, and financial milieu of a country, yet there is a shortage of resources and providers with expertise in caring for this population, particularly in underdeveloped countries around the world [8].

8. **Adolescent medicine provides an opportunity to advocate for social and political issues which directly impact the adolescents for whom we provide care.**
9. **Adolescent medicine provides an opportunity to educate future physicians and healthcare providers.**

Fellowship Training in Adolescent Medicine

Completing a fellowship in adolescent medicine is a great way to further your training in the comprehensive care of adolescent patients. The core knowledge domains expected to be covered in fellowship include preventive and general adolescent care; safety, injury, and violence; sexuality and gender; reproductive health; mental and behavioral health; substance-related issues and addictive disorders; nutrition and disordered eating; musculoskeletal health and sports medicine; endocrinology; sexually transmitted infections; ethics, legal issues, and health equity; core knowledge in scholarly activities; and general knowledge domains (i.e., the various organ systems and illnesses found in adolescent-aged patients) [9]. Adolescent medicine is a 3-year fellowship program and takes applicants that have or will have completed pediatrics, internal medicine, combined internal medicine-pediatrics, or family medicine residencies. Internal medicine and family medicine candidates may have the option to complete a 2-year rather than 3-year program and should discuss that with the programs in which they are interested.

While all fellowship programs provide training in each of the areas of the core curriculum, programs may vary in terms of what they are best known for or in which areas they provide the most exposure. For example, some programs may see many patients with teenage pregnancy and gynecological concerns, while others may see a large number of patients with eating disorders. Every program is slightly different, especially depending on the geographic location. If you have a strong interest in a particular topic, it is important to learn if the programs you are interested in will give you the exposure and training you desire in order to accomplish your academic goals.

Another great aspect about adolescent medicine is that it is often experienced directly in various sites outside of the hospital or medical office in order to meet and treat adolescent patients in their own communities. Some fellowship programs will provide opportunities to work at places such as school-based health centers, college student healthcare centers, other high schools or middle schools in the community, group homes, and juvenile justice centers. There are also different balances of outpatient versus inpatient responsibilities in each program. While adolescent medicine is largely outpatient, at some programs, adolescent physicians act as hospitalists, caring for adolescent patients that are admitted for common general medical complaints (e.g., asthma, pneumonia, and cellulitis); some programs will have an adolescent medicine inpatient admitting service for diagnosis such as pelvic inflammatory disease, abnormal uterine bleeding, or malnutrition, and some will be a consult service for similar diagnosis. It is important to choose a program where you will be satisfied with the breakdown of outpatient and inpatient roles.

When applying for adolescent medicine fellowship, just like any other residency or fellowship, location is important. You may have more time outside of the hospital than in residency, so it's helpful to be somewhere where you will be happy. However, applying broadly (if you are not geographically limited by family or other reasons) can be very helpful to give you the best chance at matching. Unlike residency, many fellowship programs only take one fellow per year (a few take two or three), so locking yourself into one geographic area or city may be more competitive, while there are many excellent programs you may love in places you might not otherwise have thought to apply. Thus, trying out a new city or state for 2 to 3 years may also allow you to explore a new place and meet new people. Receiving medical training in different regions is also a great way to learn how things may be done differently at different hospitals.

During the adolescent medicine fellowship, fellows are required to complete a scholarly activity project over the course of the period of training. Fellows will work with their fellowship program director as well as a research mentor to establish and carry out a project. Fellows are given designated protected time to work on their scholarly projects. Examples of projects that would satisfy the requirement may include a peer-reviewed publication, an in-depth manuscript, a thesis or dissertation written while completing an advanced degree, an extramural grant application, or progress reports for projects of exceptional complexity, such as a multi-year clinical trial [10, 11].

Some programs allow fellows the opportunity to obtain a Master's degree while completing fellowship. These might be a Masters of Public Health, Masters of Science, or Masters of Education, for example. You may also receive partial or full funding from your program in order to enroll and complete this degree, so this would be important to ask about if it is something you are interested in doing.

Another aspect of some programs that would be unique is if the program is designated as a Leadership in Education and Adolescent Health (LEAH) program. LEAH programs work to provide opportunities for professionals of multiple health disciplines to learn to be leaders in clinical care, research, public health policy, and advocacy in the relation to the healthcare of adolescents [12]. Regardless of LEAH designation, most programs will allow fellows many opportunities to work closely with social workers, psychologists, dietitians, and various other healthcare disciplines.

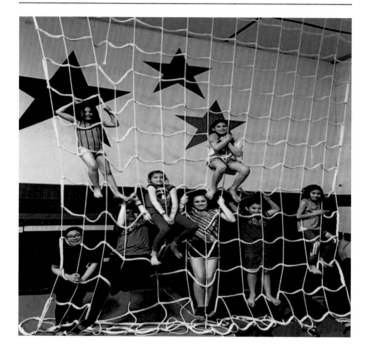

References

1. Sawyer SM, Bowes G. Adolescence on the health agenda. Lancet. 1999; 354(Suppl 2):SII31–4. https://doi.org/10.1016/s0140-6736(99)90256-8.
2. Bravender T. The foundations of interdisciplinary fellowship training in adolescent medicine in the United States. Int J Adolesc Med Health. 2016;28(3):263–7. https://doi.org/10.1515/ijamh-2016-5007.
3. Gallager JR. The origins, development, and goals of adolescent medicine. J Adolesc Health Care. 1982;3:57–63.
4. Ford CA. The role of society for adolescent health and medicine in training of health professionals. International Journal of Adolescent Medicine

and Health. 2016;28(3):339–44. http://dx.doi.org.ezaccess.libraries.psu.edu/10.1515/ijamh-2016-5020

5. Lee L, Upadhya KK, Matson PA, Adger H, Trent ME. The status of adolescent medicine: building a global adolescent workforce. Int J Adolesc Med Health. 2016;28(3):233–43. https://doi.org/10.1515/ijamh-2016-5003.

6. Butzin DW, Guerin RO, Langdon LO, Irwin CE Jr. The certification process in adolescent medicine. J Adolesc Health. 1998;23(6):328–31. https://doi.org/10.1016/s1054-139x(98)00138-4.

7. Emans SJ, Austin SB, Goodman E, Orr DP, Freeman R, Stoff D, Litt IF, Schuster MA, Haggerty R, Granger R, Irwin CE. Jr; participants of the W.T. Grant Foundation conference on Training Physician Scientists. Improving adolescent and young adult health - training the next generation of physician scientists in transdisciplinary research. J Adolesc Health. 2010;46(2):100–9. https://doi.org/10.1016/j.jadohealth.2009.10.004.

8. Golub SA, Arunakul J, Hassan A. A global perspective: training opportunities in Adolescent Medicine for healthcare professionals. Curr Opin Pediatr. 2016;28(4):447–53. https://doi.org/10.1097/MOP.0000000000000366.

9. Adolescent Medicine Content Outline. The American Board of Pediatrics. https://www.abp.org/sites/abp/files/pdf/adol_latest.pdf. 1 Jan 2020.

10. Scholarly Activity. The American Board of Pediatrics. https://www.abp.org/content/scholarly-activity.

11. Specialty-specific References for DIOs: Resident/Fellow Scholarly Activity. Accreditation Council for Graduate Medical Education (ACGME). https://www.acgme.org/Portals/0/PDFs/Specialty-specific%20Requirement%20Topics/DIO-Scholarly_Activity_Resident-Fellow.pdf. 1 July 2019.

12. LEAH Leadership Education in Adolescent Health. Health Resources & Services Administration- Maternal & Child Health. https://mchb.hrsa.gov/training/projects.asp.

Pediatric Critical Care Fellowship

3

Mary Glas Gaspers

Choosing the Right Career

I remember the moment I realized that pediatric critical care (PICU) was right for me – it was a busy PICU call night over the winter holidays during my second year of residency at AI duPont/Thomas Jefferson, and a PICU attending made a comment to me that he thought I seemed to "get it," regarding acuity, care, and treatment. That simple comment stuck with me. It made me realize that coming home after a busy PICU day was the best-feeling exhaustion I'd ever experienced. The range of ages, the physiology, the acuity, the hands-on nature of critical care, and even the difficult conversations and situations – they were right for me and my career choice.

If you're reading this chapter, you may dislike clinic days and be bored by the well child. Of course, you have fun with healthy kids, just like all pediatricians, but it's not your passion. You may strive for more continuity than you can get in the Emergency Department though you love the rapid pace of resuscitation, the anticipation of what is coming in next, and the readiness to perform needed procedures. You may be looking for more variety

M. G. Gaspers (✉)
University of Arizona, Tucson, AZ, USA
e-mail: mgaspers@peds.arizona.edu

P. M. Garrett, K. Yoon-Flannery (eds.), *A Pediatrician's Path*,
https://doi.org/10.1007/978-3-030-75370-2_3

of diagnoses or more interactive relationships with your patients than what you will find in the NICU. But critical care is only right for you if you like the whole package. There are other hands-on careers with interesting physiology, like cardiology or pulmonology, though single-organ system focus may not be your main interest. Occasionally, doctors with similar interests decide to complete anesthesia residency instead of fellowship. Critical care is not an easy path, but it is rewarding.

We in pediatric critical care have the honor and responsibility of holding a child's life in our hands, to provide the best possible resuscitative and supportive care in settings of tragedy or abuse, post heart surgery, post-transplant or during cancer care, during a severe infectious process, and in so many other complex medical situations. We practice family-centered care and take care of the child and caregiver at the same time. We have to manage the stress and emotions of parents and extended family, the needs that come with having a critically ill child.

How does one decide? Examine how you feel about the types of patients you are treating. What level of intellectual curiosity do you find in an extreme premature baby versus the range of ages found in a PICU? How do you feel about the process of rounding and the people with whom you interact? Do you enjoy the detailed yet concise systems-based approach to the PICU rounding process? Or do you prefer the rapid approach in the Emergency department – start the diagnostics de novo and triage to home or hospital? No one can decide on a career for you, and you are likely affected by family, geographical, and financial decisions. Fortunately, there are many options after training in PICU that can create a great work life and family life in your future.

Pediatrics Residency

First and foremost, PICU doctors are pediatricians. The pediatrician thinks of the future potential of their patient, not just the current situation. We think about the stages of development and safe environments for learning and growth, even while we care for their intercurrent illness. Just because you may have already identified an interest in pediatric critical care, you still owe it to yourself to become the best possible pediatrician that you can. Learn about the latest information on the disease process and treatment of your own and your coworkers' patients, examine everyone on the service, learn how to manage your time and be efficient, and learn how to develop rapport with patients and families – including how to give good and bad news with clarity and compassion. You will be expected to take and pass your boards, and the medical knowledge will only help in your further training.

Set Yourself Up for Success

Three years of residency will pass by in a flash, and there is much to learn, but in addition to the usual curriculum, there are other things that could help with critical care applications and training. It's ok if you are starting at a small residency program – PICU has a small network where people tend to know each other from their training. Get to know your PICU faculty through rotations and mentorship. Some faculty will have ongoing projects related to research or quality improvement that a resident can join – just ask to get involved. This experience can be educational as well as helpful for applications. It doesn't have to be a PICU project – any academic work will be great. Consider away rotations at other PICUs to learn about disease processes that may not be treated at your center. Also try to arrange your elective blocks to learn high-yield information. Procedural electives are fun and can build confidence, but be assured that most fellowship programs assume that you probably don't have a great deal of experience with procedures. Cardiology, pulmonology, infectious diseases, hematology/oncology, and neurology are our most common consultants, so spend some time with them during residency to learn about their approach to patients and diagnosis. Read journal articles in the critical care literature with every clinic patient – think about the treatment of the worst-case scenario in each patient you see. Still having trouble deciding? If you were sent to a remote village on a medical mission, what one journal or reference would you bring with you? What do you prefer to pick up and learn more about?

Applying for Fellowship

Fellowship for PICU involves the match, and the process involves a personal statement, a letter from your program director, and a couple faculty recommendations, as well as your choice of programs to send your application. Not all of your letters have to come from PICU faculty, but it's a good idea to have at least one from a critical care attending. Ideally, you will have a faculty member who has well-read research or is active in national committees – it's a small world and knowing people can only help. It can be a competitive match, but every year is different, depending on multiple factors. Many applicants prefer to cast a wide net, while others might be more selective geographically for family or financial reasons.

Choosing a Fellowship Program

Just like for residency, programs are accredited by the Accreditation Council for Graduate Medical Education (ACGME) and have specific educational requirements and objectives (easy to find on their website). You should consider how you learn best and what your ultimate career goals are, as well as what your interests are for research and patient types. Large programs (>1500 admissions/year) are heavy on experience, with less time for thinking and reading; medium programs (1000–1500 admissions/year) are a mix of seeing and doing; small programs (<1000 admissions/year) will require extra reading but may also have less fellows to compete for experience and procedures. Ultimately, if the program is ACGME-approved, you will get a good training.

Talk to recent residency graduates that went on to fellowship. How do the PICU fellows like working at that center? Keep in mind: if you ask a marathon runner (during the race) when their next marathon will be, they might just spit in your face. So, with a grain of salt, ask objectively – are they learning, are they doing procedures, are they teaching, do they have research opportunities, are their colleagues supportive, or is there mentorship? The answer to all of that is probably yes. Ultimately, all of the guidelines and hands-on time will allow you to be ready for PICU attendingness, no matter where you go. Pick the brains of your faculty about programs you should consider, then research them on their websites. All of the legwork will allow for better questions during your interview process.

During your interviews, you will again need to have some goals and interests in mind. Research is a big part of your 3 years, so having a research interest to talk about will be a plus. Programs will be looking for applicants that have common interests and clearly defined goals, with a clear reason for applying to their program.

During Fellowship

Eat when you can, drink when you can, pee when you can, and sleep when you can. Lean on your friends and mentors and provide that support right back when you can. Brace yourself, because the training can be intense. You may want to quit, maybe in the middle of a shift or after a tough code. I went through this and got to the other side by remembering *why* I chose PICU in the first place. Fortunately, most children will do well after a critical illness, and you are passionate about this goal to help support them and get them playing again. Academic centers that have fellowship programs will be high-volume, high-acuity, quaternary centers of critical care pediatrics, and you will see kids die. News flash: it doesn't get easier as you get older. You will always question your decisions when the outcome is bad – this is part of being a good doctor. No one knows everything and you cannot improve without self-reflection. If you did the best for the patient and they still die, you can carry their family through the process and make a difference even in death. You learn to cope and learn more every day as you practice your art of medicine.

In order to succeed in fellowship, start with a broad knowledge of pediatrics and a working knowledge of when procedures are needed. You will need to read a ton – background information to start, and then recent published guidelines and ongoing research into a topic. Experience as much learning as you can and work hard (within the allowed work hours) while at work. Then go home and have some fun; exercise; participate in your spiritual life; read a fun book; keep in contact with partners, family, and friends; and be a normal person. Allow the mind to relax. Let me be a mom here – also try to eat healthy, minimize alcohol, sleep enough, wear your seatbelt, and don't text while driving.

Looking for a Critical Care Job

Look how amazing you are! You survived the rigorous schedule of PICU fellowship, and now you get to apply for an attending job. Academic or private? Rural or urban? The world is your oyster. Local economic output of any given city, existing faculty complement and patient census/demographics, among other factors, will determine who is hiring. Talk to recent graduates about what to expect and have your career goals solidly in mind when you go to interview. The Society of Critical Care Medicine (SCCM) posts a list of centers that are hiring, and it's also ok to email the PICU physician leader to express your interest even if they haven't advertised a position. On the interview trail, be ready to ask questions about clinical schedule, expectations for nonclinical time, how to be promoted, how consultants work with PICU, and any questions you have about research, teaching, or anything else. You want to be happy where you are, since the work will still be rigorous. Lifelong learning is essential in pediatric critical care medicine, and you are lucky to be involved in a continuously growing and expanding field – this is one of the attractive attributes of pediatric critical care medicine.

Part of your critical care career could involve research, and mine has involved participation in Pediatric Acute Lung Injury and Sepsis Investigators (PALISI) for clinical research projects. Three of my friends from fellowship and I have enjoyed this collaboration together, especially the bi-annual conferences. We are pictured here in New Orleans in March 2020 enjoying beignets during a break. I'm the one on the right. Lifelong learning and lifelong friendships have been a nice side effect of my rigorous fellowship in pediatric critical care, and I hope you also find your passion. Thanks to Simi Jeyapalan, DO, for her thoughts about this chapter – she's in the flowered shirt below. Also pictured are Shira Gertz, MD (left), and Katri Typpo, MD MPH (right center).

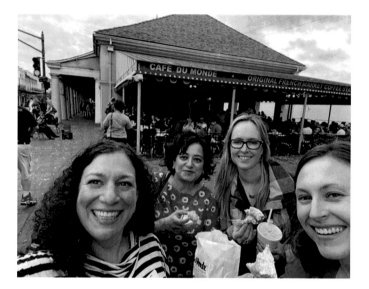

Pediatric Emergency Medicine Fellowship

4

Lauren A. McNickle
and Robert P. Olympia

A Brief History of Pediatric Emergency Medicine (PEM)

The field of PEM originated in the 1970s, when discussions regarding the optimization of care for critically ill and injured infants and children began among general pediatricians. The goal of PEM was to improve and ensure the quality of patient care, teaching, and research in this new field of pediatric medicine. In the 1980s, sections of PEM were established in the American Academy of Pediatrics (AAP) and American College of Emergency Physicians (ACEP). The 1980s also introduced specialized certification for the management of critically ill and injured infants and children [including Pediatric Advanced Life Support (PALS), a module for injured children in Advanced Trauma Life Support (ATLS), and Advanced Pediatric Life Support (APLS)] and the first PEM-dedicated journal, "Pediatric Emergency Care."

L. A. McNickle
Department of Emergency Medicine, Baystate Medical Center,
Springfield, MA, USA
e-mail: lauren.mcnickle@baystatehealth.org,
lmcnickle@pennstatehealth.psu.edu

R. P. Olympia (✉)
Department of Emergency Medicine & Pediatrics, Penn State Hershey
Medical Center, Hershey, PA, USA
e-mail: rolympia@hmc.psu.edu

© The Author(s), under exclusive license to Springer Nature
Switzerland AG 2021
P. M. Garrett, K. Yoon-Flannery (eds.), *A Pediatrician's Path*,
https://doi.org/10.1007/978-3-030-75370-2_4

The dissemination of PEM research is well represented at both regional and national scientific assemblies, including the AAP National Conference & Exhibition, Pediatric Academic Societies (PAS) meeting, ACEP Scientific Assembly, and Society for Academic Emergency Medicine (SAEM) meeting. Research in the field of PEM is often published in high-impact factor journals, most recently including topics such as pain management, asthma, procedural sedation, bronchiolitis, ultrasound, resuscitation, and simulation [1].

Pediatric emergency departments (PEDs) were first described in the 1960s. Currently, 70% of PEDs are located in large urban areas affiliated with or located within university teaching hospitals, with 50% of the PEDs population under the age of 3 years and the greatest pediatric volume presenting to the PED between 3 pm and midnight. While most PEDs are prepared to manage the acutely ill or injured infant or child, often presenting with respiratory distress, abnormal mental status, abnormal rhythm or perfusion, ingestions/poisonings, and acute surgical conditions, the most common PEDs diagnoses are acute febrile illness, acute respiratory illness, otitis media, viral infection, and asthma exacerbation, and the most common diagnoses in adolescents are acute headache, nonspecific abdominal pain, and psychiatric-related complaint [2].

So Why Should You Choose a Career in PEM?

1. *Organized chaos.* The fast-paced atmosphere with a variety of ages and chief complaints hits you like a hurricane. Every day is a different day, making for an exciting career. If you dislike the monotony of inpatient rounding, then PEM is perfect for you. PEM physicians are frontline diagnosticians, under time constraints to solve each undifferentiated patient that comes through the door. We love the adrenaline rush.
2. *Flexibility.* Often you can choose how many shifts you work per month, days or nights, and weekdays or weekends. On average, PEM physicians work 10.6 shifts a month that are 8.9 hours in duration. When looking at the total hours per week, PEM physicians work 26.7 hours fulfilling clinical duties and 42.7 when accounting for all clinical and nonclinical responsibilities [3]. Bunch your ED shifts up for an instant vacation. Purely work clinical ED shifts, or add research,

education, and administration to your responsibilities. The PEM world is your oyster.

3. *Location, location, location.* In the past, most PEM attending positions were located in urban areas affiliated with academic institutions. Not anymore. Since many community hospitals and academic institutions are opting to have PEDs staffed by board-certified specialists, PEM physicians can be more selective on where to establish their careers.

4. *A career of scholarship.* The volume of patients, the variety of disease processes, and new technologies and innovations in the field of PEM, such as simulation, ultrasound, and point-of-care diagnostic testing, allow the PEM physician a multitude of opportunities to perform research and quality improvement projects, with the goal of promotion and improving the care of children.

5. *The jack of all trades, the master of many.* One minute, you are the pediatric surgeon running a traumatic resuscitation and placing a chest tube, and the next minute you are the anesthesiologist intubating a postoperative congenital heart infant. Procedural sedations, fracture reductions and casting, lumbar punctures, complex laceration repairs, and central venous lines are some of the procedures we routinely perform. Complex medical patients and acutely ill or injured surgical patients are some of those we care for. The variety of patients and procedures is exhilarating.

6. *The ultimate team sport.* Whether it's a cardiorespiratory arrest or a traumatic resuscitation, status epilepticus or septic shock, or nonurgent chief complaints, the success of your patients depends on an entire team working as a synchronous unit. Resident physicians and medical students, PED nurses and technicians, registration and environmental services, diagnostic and laboratory technicians, social workers, chaplains, transport, child life, and subspecialty services all need to work hand-in-hand. And the PEM physician is the coach of the team.

7. *Get out in the community and serve.* Whether it's injury prevention, school-based health, emergency and disaster preparedness or community education on immunizations, gun violence, teen distracted driving, alcohol/drug abuse, or bullying, PEM physicians feel an innate desire to impart knowledge to the community it serves. It's about making a difference in the lives of children.

8. *Gaining acceptance is our challenge.* Parents bring their children to the PED, usually stressed, fearful, and vulnerable. They are often unfamiliar with those who will make, at times, life-saving decisions on behalf of their loved ones. We must listen attentively, communicate clearly, and gain their trust unconditionally. It is a challenge that we as PEM physicians accept willingly.

9. *The PEM family is tight.* Whether it's scanning the medical literature, running into PEM colleagues at conferences and scientific assemblies, or listening to social media podcasts or webcasts, PEM physicians are well represented. We are a small, tight-knit community, where everyone knows your name. We work hard and play hard, and we have fun fighting as a united front for the health and wellness of infants and children.

10. *Money doesn't buy happiness, but it sure does help.* Financial compensation is on the higher end compared with other pediatric subspecialties, and if you work within a Department of Emergency Medicine, your salary may be comparable to other general EM physicians.

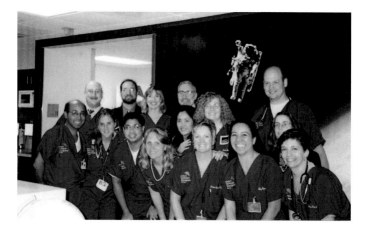

Photo of emergency medicine colleagues during Dr. Olympia's first year of PEM fellowship, Children's Hospital at Montefiore, Bronx, NY

PEM Fellowship: The Next Steps

PEM certification requires the completion of a 3-year fellowship for pediatric residency graduates and 2-year fellowship for emergency medicine residency graduates, often the completion of a research and quality improvement requirement, and the passing of an initial PEM board certification examination, followed by subsequent PEM recertification examinations.

There are currently 81 PEM fellowship programs in the United States, with 199 first-year positions offered in the 2019 match [4]. In addition to ED shifts in the PED and general ED, rotations may include critical care, anesthesia, trauma, toxicology, orthopedics, child abuse, pre-hospital care, OB/GYN, transport medicine, general surgery and other surgical subspecialties, radiology, ultrasound, simulation, and global health. Complementing medical and surgical topics, didactic curriculum often includes topics on research and quality improvement, administration and business, and teaching and education.

Based on data from the National Resident Matching Program (NRMP), PEM is considered one of the most competitive fellowships within the field of pediatrics. For applicants in the 2019–2020 PEM fellowship pool, the match rate was 77.1%; the match rate for other pediatric subspecialties exceeded 90% [4]. Although these numbers may seem daunting, do not let these statistics deter you from your desire to pursue a career in PEM. With strategic planning, one can work to create an exceptional application.

Paramount to the PEM application process is building your curriculum vitae (CV). Search for opportunities that mirror your professional interests (what areas of PEM are you really passionate about?): (1) Seek out educational opportunities at your medical school, residency, or even outside your institution (other nonpediatric residency programs, grand rounds at other institutions, or with community outreach programs). Turn every lecture into a review article or book chapter. (2) Get involved in research and quality improvement opportunities, but choose projects that you can complete during the first 2 years of residency, usually during less stressful rotations. Consider taking research electives to collect and analyze data, and write up abstracts and manuscripts. Retrospective studies and case reports work well within your time constraints. Turn every research and quality improvement project into a lecture, an abstract to present at a regional or national scientific assembly, and a peer-reviewed journal manuscript submission. (3) Participate in committees within your residency program, your hospital and institution, your medical school, your profession (such as AAP, PAS, ACEP, or SAEM), and your community. Demonstrate leadership and ability to work within a team structure.

Another important requirement for the PEM application are letters of recommendation (LOR). Similar to medical school, you want to find LOR writers who know you well [professionally (can comment on your clinical acumen, research and teaching abilities, service) and personally, if possible] and can write a strong letter on your behalf. Most PEM fellowships require 3–4 LORs, often one from your residency program director, at least one from a PEM attending physician, and at least one from a pediatric critical care attending. LOR writers who have connections to your top PEM choices will often improve your chances of success. If you are fortunate to be able to do an away PEM elective, attempt to obtain a LOR from a senior attending who can accumulate the comments from the physicians you worked with. In addition to LORs, having physicians from your institution contact PEM programs that you are interested in will benefit you in the long run. As the saying goes, sometimes it's who you know in addition to what you know.

The final step to a well-rounded PEM fellowship application includes a personal statement. Trying to describe yourself in words can be very difficult. As it is a personal statement, each individual's story will be unique. PEM faculty already appreciate the field of PEM, so focus your personal statement on traits that make you a unique candidate, highlighting things on your CV that you were truly passionate about and on what that program should expect from you during fellowship and beyond. Sell yourself, be honest, and let your words shine through.

As you begin to put your application together, it is also important to begin considering the programs you will apply to. On average, most applicants apply to approximately ten programs; however, this may vary by applicant circumstance [5]. When selecting programs, consider what is important to you: location, fellowship size, research opportunities, teaching/supervisory responsibilities, advanced degree opportunities, moonlighting opportunities, etc. The American Academy of Medical Colleges (AAMC) website provides resources on applying for fellowship, a list of fellowships, and links to the Electronic Residency Application Service (ERAS) with deadlines for applications. Undertaking the process of applying to a PEM fellowship can be confusing and overwhelming at times. Remember to reach out to your mentors regularly throughout residency to help guide and encourage you along your pathway to success.

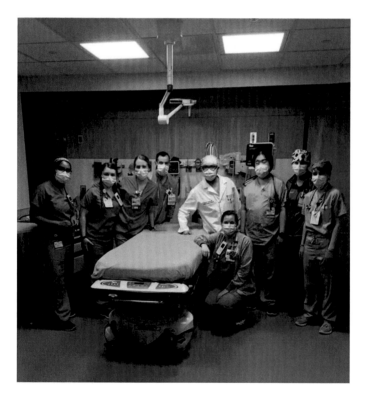

Dr. Olympia (orange cap) and Dr. McNickle (yellow cap) waiting for a pediatric resuscitation, Penn State Hershey Children's Hospital, Hershey, PA

References

1. Spurkeland N, Rixe J, Glick J, Lehman E, Olympia RP. Publishing trends in the field of pediatric emergency medicine from 2004-2013. Pediatr Emerg Care. 2016;32(12):840–5.
2. Alpern ER, Stanley RM, Gorelick MH, Donaldson A, Knight S, Teach SJ, Singh T, Mahajan P, Goepp JG, Kuppermann N, Dean JM, Chamberlain JM. Pediatric Emergency Care Applied Research Network (PECARN). Epidemiology of a pediatric emergency medicine research network: The PECARN Core Data Project. Pediatr Emerg Care. 2006;22(10):689–99.
3. Gorelick MH, Schremmer R, Ruch-Ross C, Radabaugh C, Selbst S. Current workforce characteristics and burnout in pediatric emergency medicine. Academic Emerg Med. 2016;23(1):48–54.
4. National Resident Matching Program. National Resident Matching Program, Results and Data: Specialties Matching Service 2020 Appointment Year. [Internet]. Washington, DC: National Resident Matching Program; 2020 [updated 2020 Feb; cited 2020 Jun 6] Available from: https://mk0nrmp3oyqui6wqfm.kinstacdn.com/wp-content/uploads/2020/02/Results-and-Data-SMS-2020.pdf.
5. Wall J, Ford CJ. Pediatric emergency medicine [Internet]. Irving, TX: Emergency Medicine Residents' Association; 2018. [Cited 2020 Jun 9]. Available from: https://www.emra.org/books/fellowship-guide-book/19-pediatric-em/.

Pediatric Endocrinology Fellowship

5

Andrew Palladino

Overview

A fellowship in Pediatric Endocrinology is 3 years in length, and applicants must complete a residency in Pediatrics or Medicine/ Pediatrics prior to starting fellowship. The majority of Pediatric Endocrinology fellowship programs accept applications through Electronic Residency Application Service (ERAS) and participate in a match conducted through the National Resident Matching Program (NRMP). For information on participating programs and timelines, applicants should visit the Association of American Medical Colleges (AAMC) and NRMP websites. Applicants should contact nonparticipating fellowship programs directly to inquire about their application process.

A fellowship in Pediatric Endocrinology will provide training in the management of general endocrine disorders (growth, thyroid, puberty, pituitary gland, adrenal glands, parathyroid glands) and diabetes. Additionally, some pediatric endocrine programs may be referral centers for more rare endocrine conditions (e.g., hyperinsulinism, ambiguous genitalia) due to the presence of expertise in multiple pediatric specialties at the institution. Fellowship programs vary in size from one to four fellows per year and are affiliated with either a freestanding academic chil-

A. Palladino (✉)
Pfizer, Inc., Collegeville, PA, USA

© The Author(s), under exclusive license to Springer Nature Switzerland AG 2021
P. M. Garrett, K. Yoon-Flannery (eds.), *A Pediatrician's Path*,
https://doi.org/10.1007/978-3-030-75370-2_5

35

dren's hospital or as part of a pediatric department in a university hospital or medical center. Typically, the first year is dedicated to clinical training, while the second and third years are focused on research training in either patient-oriented or basic laboratory research. However, program curricula may vary allowing for greater focus on clinical training in the second and third years. This may be an important difference when considering programs, depending on whether you want a more clinically or research-focused fellowship experience. Keep in mind that all programs consist of a research training component and an ACGME-required scholarly project in order to graduate from the program. Trainees in most programs will also have a weekly endocrine continuity clinic throughout their 3 years of training.

Some programs will expect their trainees to participate in a small research project during their first year of training and even submit an abstract for a poster presentation at a national meeting during their first year of fellowship. Most programs will expect their trainees to present their research at a national meeting, either as a poster or as an oral presentation, sometime during their second or third year of fellowship.

Some fellowship programs require trainees to apply for grant funding to support their salary during the third year of fellowship. If one is unable to secure their own funding, programs will usually find a way to fund the fellow, but it is important to ask a program how their second and third year trainees are funded, if you need to secure your own funding, and what happens if you don't successfully do so.

In addition to what is mentioned above, when considering the type of program you are looking for, it is important to consider whether you want a busy, subspecialized endocrine division with a large research focus (e.g., a division with a diabetes center, a thyroid center, a bone center, etc.) versus a smaller clinically focused program. It is essential to understand the impact that the size of the institution will have and what the mix of inpatient and outpatient care will be. Programs in larger tertiary and quaternary care centers will provide more exposure to complex endocrine patients with comorbid conditions and higher acuity, but it will also mean more time receiving inpatient training (>50% of your first year will be spent on inpatient and consult services) compared to smaller programs where more of the focus may be in outpatient care. The difference in these settings may also impact the quantity and quality of in-house and telephone calls you will take as a fellow.

All clinics and hospitals will provide interesting patients and the necessary training as described, but the volume, acuity, and complexity will likely vary between the smaller and larger programs. The other major difference lies in the research opportunities that are available at different programs. One of the most important things you can do when researching fellowship programs is to find out what past fellows have gone on to do after fellowship. A program may boast about their research program, but if none of the fellows in the past 5 years have gone into research, that is a red flag if a research career is your goal. If you are looking for a clinical program but the majority of former fellows continue doing predominantly research after training, that may not be the program for you. If you are unsure whether or not you want to do research after fellowship, it is probably in your best interest to find a program that offers strong research training but has a good balance of graduates that have gone on to do both clinical work and research. Obviously, if you already have an idea of what area you would like to do research in, you should focus on programs and investigators or universities that would meet your needs.

Applying

A strong applicant for a Pediatric Endocrinology fellowship is someone who has shown a continued interest in Pediatric Endocrinology. One way to do this is by completing an elective rotation in endocrine at your home institution. Other ways are by being involved in the writing of a paper related to pediatric endocrinology or by being part of a research project related to pediatric endocrinology. If these opportunities are not available in endocrinology, they should be sought out in other areas in order to demonstrate your willingness to collaborate and your desire to learn beyond what the basic rotations of residency offer.

If you can, it's best to do an elective rotation as a resident at one of the programs that you are interested in. This is a great way to see what it would be like to be a fellow at that program as well as get to know the current fellows and gauge their attitudes about the program. This is also a good opportunity for the program to get to know you and your chance to make a great impression. You will want to do everything you can to function at the level of a fellow so that they can picture you in that role. Make sure to get all of your questions answered while you are there and to get a feel not just for the endocrine division but the rest of the hospital and other subspecialties, as you will be working with other divisions and departments within the hospital.

In preparing your application for fellowship, you should get letters of recommendation from attending physicians that can speak to your character, patient care abilities, and medical knowledge. You should ask any attendings that you have worked with on research projects or papers to write you a letter of recommendation. If possible, you should get a letter of recommendation from one of the endocrine attendings from your home hospital or away elective endocrine rotation.

Interviews

Once you've selected the programs you're going to apply to, it's time to prepare for the interviews. The faculty and fellows that will interview you want to get a sense of whether or not you will "fit in" at their program, just as you should be using the interview day to see if you think the program is a good fit for you. No one is going to quiz you on your endocrine knowledge. They are only going to ask you what you already know, so relax. You should be prepared for questions about your reason for choosing a career in Pediatric Endocrinology and about any research you have done or any papers/presentations you have on your CV. You should prepare ahead of time and know who the faculty members are at the program where you are interviewing and where their clinical or research interests lie. Be prepared to have questions for the interviewers; they are going to want to know what questions you have about the program. Most programs will host a dinner the night before the interview that is just for the applicants and fellows. You should definitely attend this dinner to get to know the other fellows. It is also an opportunity for the fellows to get to know you, which they can't really do on the interview day, and many programs solicit feedback from their fellows regarding the applicants. Once you have completed your interviews, you will have to create your rank list based upon which programs you're most interested and which fit best with your life circumstances. You will find out where you have matched about 6 months prior to starting fellowship.

During and After Fellowship

At some point during your fellowship training, you will make a decision as to whether you want to primarily see patients after fellowship or if you want to pursue a research career. This is an important decision because after fellowship your salary needs to come from somewhere, and it will either be generated from seeing patients or from research grant funding.

Fellows that go on to clinical practice may stay on at the same institution, depending on the availability of clinical positions, or may move on to another institution. It will depend on a number of factors such as where the fellow wants to live, job availability in the area, and salary. A clinical position typically involves 3.5 to 4.5 days of clinic per week, with the remaining time protected as administrative (nonclinical) time. Most often, fellows that do research after training stay on at the institution at which they trained because their mentor and research project are there. They may get small grants, plus some funding from their mentor, and work 1 to 2 days in the clinic to fund their time, while they continue to work on their research in preparation to eventually get a large enough grant to fund all of their time. It often takes several years after training to secure significant grant funding and not everyone is able to do this.

After training, in addition to being a Pediatric Endocrinologist who sees patients or does research or both, there are opportunities to be involved in medical student, resident, and fellow education. You may also have the chance to be involved in quality improvement work or for leadership positions at the divisional and departmental levels within the hospital or institution. Additionally, there is also the option to enter the pharmaceutical industry following the completion of your fellowship or anytime thereafter, though having a few years of clinical experience can be quite beneficial. There are a number of pharmaceutical companies involved in the development and marketing of endocrine and diabetes therapeutics who are recruiting pediatric endocrinologists with clinical research experience.

After 3 years you will complete your endocrine fellowship, and you will get out of it what you have put into it, regardless of where you have trained. After fellowship you need to do what will make you happy, not what will make you money. Pediatric endocrinologists aren't in it for the money, we enjoy the diseases, the treatments, the research, and our patients.

Pediatric Gastroenterology Fellowship

6

Elizabeth C Maxwell

Introduction

Pediatric gastroenterology (GI) is an exciting field of digestive functions and the diseases that affect them in children. We take care of babies who spit up, preschoolers who are constipated and withholding stool, children who aren't growing, and adolescents with chronic abdominal pain. We diagnose and treat chronic diseases including celiac disease, inflammatory bowel disease (Crohn's disease and ulcerative colitis), eosinophilic esophagitis (EoE), functional GI disorders, and motility disorders. We take care of patients with acute liver dysfunction, some of whom go on to require liver transplant. Our field includes an enjoyable mix of outpatient visits, inpatient care, and procedures.

If You Are Still in Residency and Even Remotely Considering GI

The North American Society of Pediatric Gastroenterology, Hepatology, and Nutrition (NASPGHAN), which is our specialty's organization dedicated to advancing research, education, and

E. C. Maxwell (✉)
Department of Pediatrics, Perelman School of Medicine, University of Pennsylvania, Philadelphia, PA, USA
e-mail: maxwelle@email.chop.edu

© The Author(s), under exclusive license to Springer Nature Switzerland AG 2021
P. M. Garrett, K. Yoon-Flannery (eds.), *A Pediatrician's Path*, https://doi.org/10.1007/978-3-030-75370-2_6

clinical practice in pediatric GI, hosts a special program for pediatric residents interested in GI fellowship at our annual meeting, called the Teaching and Tomorrow Program. It is a wonderful opportunity to see first-hand the exciting basic, translational, and clinical research updates in the field and to experience the community of pediatric GI physicians who gather from across the USA and worldwide for this annual meeting. Specifically, the Teaching and Tomorrow Program participants attend the postgraduate course, poster sessions, and any of the plenaries and concurrent sessions they would like during the meeting. There are also smaller special events for Teaching and Tomorrow Program participants to learn about GI fellowship and the application and interview process, including a reception with current GI fellows and fellowship program directors. Typically, pediatric residents attend this meeting in the fall of their PL-2 year.

GI Fellowship Training Programs

There are 64 pediatric GI training programs in the USA [1]. Program size varies from one to five fellows per year, and the fellowship length is 3 years. Currently, pediatric GI is part of the July subspecialty timeline for ERAS, with applications submitted in July, interviews occurring in the fall, and the match taking place in December during the third year of pediatric residency [2]. The 3 years of fellowship include clinical training and completion of a scholarly project, with procedural training occurring throughout. The NASPGHAN training guidelines recommend 15–24 months of clinical training and 12–21 months dedicated to completion of scholarly work [3].

There is some flexibility in training elements, depending on individual fellow career interests as well as areas of expertise within training programs, pediatric GI divisions, and hospitals, to allow for each fellow's training experience to best prepare him or her for the next step in his or her career. For example, there are some research training grants for fellows that limit their clinical time during the latter part of fellowship. Fellows who participate in clinical research and are planning for a clinical career post-fellowship may broaden and add to their clinical responsibilities to include extra training in certain areas, such as intestinal failure, hepatology, nutrition, motility, pancreatology, or inflammatory bowel disease (IBD), to name a few. In addition, there are some formal 1-year advanced fellowships available including transplant hepatology, inflammatory bowel disease, nutrition, and advanced endoscopy.

Clinical Training

A significant portion of clinical training in pediatric GI fellowship occurs in the inpatient setting. Depending on the size of the program and institution, there is often a GI inpatient service as well as a GI consult service. There may be a separate service for hepatology and liver transplant patients. However, clinical pediatric GI is predominantly an outpatient specialty, and the training guidelines recommend devoting a significant portion of clinical training during fellowship to the ambulatory setting as well. One half day of outpatient continuity clinic throughout the 3 years is recommended, and fellows who are headed toward a clinical career will likely do more [3].

The American Board of Pediatrics (ABP) outlines specifications for content that you will learn as a pediatric GI fellow (Table 6.1). Beyond these topics, the content specifications for the board exam also outline in more detail disorders of each area of the GI tract: mouth, esophagus, stomach, small bowel, large bowel, liver, pancreas, bile ducts, and gallbladder. Pediatric GI fellowship training also includes nutrition, motility, psychosocial, and ethical considerations [4].

Endoscopy and Other Procedures: A Picture (and Some Biopsies!) Is Worth a Thousand Words

Pediatric GI is a procedural subspecialty. Our primary procedures include esophagogastroduodenoscopy (EGD) and colonoscopy. Visual examination of the mucosa and histological data from

Table 6.1 Highlights of the ABP Board Content Specifications for pediatric GI [4]

Common GI topics	GI signs and symptoms: pathophysiology
· Functional constipation and encopresis	· Failure to thrive
· Celiac disease	· Vomiting and regurgitation
· Short bowel syndrome	· Acute abdominal pain
· Functional GI disorders	· Chronic abdominal pain
· Inflammatory bowel disease	· Colic and gas
· Eosinophilic esophagitis	· Diarrhea
· *Helicobacter pylori* infection	· Malabsorption
· Gastroesophageal reflux and esophagitis	· Gastrointestinal bleeding
· Nonalcoholic fatty liver disease	· Abdominal mass
· Autoimmune hepatitis	· Jaundice
· Pancreatitis	· Liver failure
· Parenteral nutrition	· Dysphagia
	· Hepatomegaly
	· Ascites

mucosal biopsies which we send to our pathologists help us diagnose celiac disease, Crohn's disease, ulcerative colitis, eosinophilic esophagitis, and *Helicobacter pylori* gastritis, among others. More advanced procedures include foreign body removal, polypectomy, balloon dilation, and control of bleeding using various endoscopic techniques. We also perform percutaneous liver biopsy and paracentesis. Our procedures are routine in certain clinical scenarios, but there are a few GI procedural emergencies including esophageal button battery retrieval, examinations following caustic ingestions, and controlling brisk upper GI bleeds. Endoscopy is fun to learn, and skills improve with experience (and with guidance from experienced faculty), so the more you do, the better you will get!

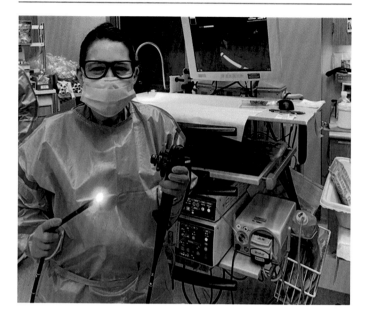

Scholarship

All GI fellows must participate in basic, clinical, or translational research, or another scholarly activity during fellowship. This project ideally is begun or planned during the first year of training and completed by the end of fellowship. Mentorship is incredibly important to guide fellows through this process. In addition to the specific project you will work on with your mentor (studying a model of biliary atresia in a basic science lab, analysis of stool samples for a particular biomarker associated with bacterial overgrowth, describing early outcomes for pediatric IBD patients started on a new biologic therapy), you will also learn biostatistics, epidemiology, basic and clinical laboratory research methodology and study design, and how to apply research to clinical practice. Lastly, you will learn the skills of communication of your scholarship in both written (submit your manuscript to Journal of Pediatric Gastroenterology and Nutrition (JPGN)!) and oral forms (oral presentation at the NASPGHAN annual meeting!) [3].

What Will Make Me a Successful Applicant for Pediatric GI Fellowship?

Programs are looking for a commitment to the field, including past experiences within clinical and research areas, as well as some ideas about your career goals within pediatric GI. Perhaps you are interested in becoming a pediatric transplant hepatologist and have participated in a research project related to cholestasis in infants. Or maybe you took care of a patient on inpatient general pediatrics who came in with weight loss and bloody diarrhea who was diagnosed with inflammatory bowel disease, and you are planning to work with a physician in your program's IBD center on therapeutic drug monitoring of biologic agents in your IBD patient population. Many successful applicants have participated in basic science research at the time they apply for fellowship, but this is not a requirement. Program directors recognize that your fellowship training years will be the time that you will refine your career interests and goals within the field. It is important, however, that you have demonstrated your passion to learn more about pediatric GI in some way – basic science or translational research, clinical research, quality improvement, advocacy, medical education – and that you highlight these experiences in your application and during interviews.

How Do I Choose the Program That's Right for Me?

NASPGHAN training guidelines and the American College of Graduate Medical Education (ACGME) have ensured that each accredited pediatric GI fellowship program will meet the requirements to train competent pediatric gastroenterologists. There are, however, differences in programs that will shape the experience and training of the fellows. Besides the factors that would apply to any fellowship program variety (such as location), there are some GI-specific variables to consider. The size of the program will influence the clinical demands as well as exposure to both straightforward ("bread and butter") GI cases and very rare disorders (the "zebras"). Programs that have subspecialty centers (IBD, liver transplant, motility) may provide you with more in-depth exposure to certain areas within GI. The research interests of current faculty will impact and influence your research opportunities. Often there is collaboration with adult GI colleagues for educational sessions, conferences, and research opportunities. Don't forget about the related specialties that are important for GI – our pathologists, radiologists, surgeons, dieticians, social workers, and psychologists are essential to providing excellent GI care. Lastly, the interactions during your interview day with the faculty, fellows, and the hospital environment will go a long way to helping you decide which program is the best fit.

References

1. Pediatric Gastroenterology (Pediatrics). Available from: https://services. aamc.org/eras/erasstats/par/display.cfm?NAV_ROW=PAR&SPEC_ CD=332.
2. Match calendars. Available from: https://www.nrmp.org/match-calendars/.
3. Leichtner AM, Gillis LA, Gupta S, Heubi J, Kay M, Narkewicz MR, et al. NASPGHAn Guidelines for Training in Pediatric Gastroenterology. JPGN. 2013;56:S1–S38.
4. The American Board of Pediatrics. Content Outline for Subspecialties. Available from: https://www.abp.org/apply-exam/about-our-certifying-exams/content-outlines-subspecialties.

Pediatric Infectious Diseases Fellowship

7

Amol Purandare

Introduction

Infectious diseases (ID) is a dynamic and exciting field of medicine. ID providers are one of the few specialists consulted in every area of the hospital and clinic settings. They must be knowledgeable regarding conditions affecting patients prenatally and beyond. From common diseases to pandemics, ID specialists play an important role in staying informed and interfacing with providers, administration, and the public. The field is flexible in career options after fellowship and compared to other specialties can allow for a more desirable work-life balance. A pediatric infectious diseases fellowship is a 3-year training program at a designated institution.

Starting Out

If you have an initial interest in pediatric ID, there are a few steps you should take before the application process. The first step is finding a mentor. It is helpful to find an ID physician at your

A. Purandare (✉)
Pediatric Infectious Diseases, Children's Mercy Hospital,
Kansas City, MO, USA
e-mail: Avpurandare@cmh.edu

© The Author(s), under exclusive license to Springer Nature
Switzerland AG 2021
P. M. Garrett, K. Yoon-Flannery (eds.), *A Pediatrician's Path*,
https://doi.org/10.1007/978-3-030-75370-2_7

institution or another that can discuss the field with you. You can ask non-ID mentors if they have an acquaintance in the field that would be able to talk in person, by phone, or via email. Hearing about the field can be a big step in figuring out if it is right for you. Another initial step to take is looking into the Pediatric Infectious Diseases Society (PIDS); it is a wonderful resource for learning more about fellowship training and careers. Browsing the society website at PIDS.org can give an idea of current society activities, career and grant opportunities, as well as a complete list of training programs under the Education and Training section. Residents can join PIDS, which can help foster relationships, inform about conferences, and find connections to potential fellowships.

Know Your Interests

Once you have decided that infectious diseases is the field for you, the next step is determining if you have any early interests to help shape your training and eventually, your career. In addition to caring for general infectious diseases patients, most infectious diseases physicians also have other duties and areas of focus. While not necessary before starting fellowship, finding a niche can help guide your career path and help determine if a fellowship location fits you. For example, you may have a research focus looking at a specific organism, disease state, or quality improvement. Many pediatric ID centers were started with an emphasis on Special Immunology, which focuses primarily on HIV-exposed and HIV-infected patients. There is a growing presence of specialists participating in immunocompromised and transplant care. Antimicrobial stewardship is a requirement in hospitals, with ID physicians and pharmacists being the leaders. ID providers tend to be the backbone of hospital infection prevention programs. You may find ID to be complementary to global health endeavors as well.

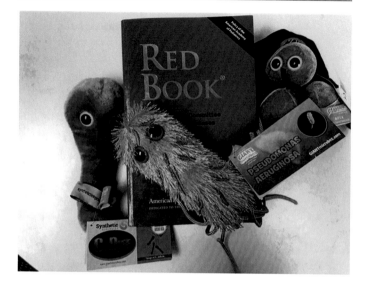

What to Look for in Programs

Choosing a potential fellowship program occurs next. While you will get quality training and be taught the same core principles across all accredited Infectious Diseases fellowship programs, it is important to know that not all programs are the same. There are multiple factors to consider when determining if the training program is right for you. Even if a program is well established or recognized in other fields, it may not mean it is the program that will meet your learning and career goals. First, you should determine if the location of the program is a place you can see yourself living. Unlike other fields, there tends to be good availability of pediatric ID training positions across the nation. It is important to make sure you will be happy living in a city and feel that you have adequate support. You should look into the structure of the program and your overall training, and discuss with your mentor if the program is a good fit. Factors to look into are the time spent on inpatient service, outpatient clinic time, exposure to immunocompromised patients, and special immunology training. Understanding patient load, and if a program's current structure is dependent on fellows or not, can be important when determining your own learning style, ability to balance work/life responsibilities, and feeling as you have obtained adequate patient care experience. If you do have a niche in mind already, see if there is a potential mentor or learning experience at the program you're seeking. Finally, programs may have more appeal to you if they offer unique or additional opportunities during your training such as dynamic antimicrobial stewardship programs (ASPs), prospects of working with particular mentors or lab setting, opportunities to pursue additional degrees, experiences at public health or regulatory bodies, or dedicated global health elective time.

Fellowship Application and Interviews

Application for pediatric infectious diseases fellowship is through Electronic Residency Application Service (ERAS), currently on the July application schedule. A list of participating programs for the application year can be found on the ERAS website. Occasionally programs may have spots not present on the application cycle. These may be advertised on the PIDS website or can at times be found on career listing sites. Applicants with VISAs should check with programs prior to applying. Applicants should consider applying to multiple programs. Programs have different feels in their clinical duties, research opportunities, and nonclinical opportunities. Interviews tend to be fairly flexible in scheduling, and coordinators can work with you in determining the best times to interview. It is important when scheduling interviews to let programs know of specific interests or if there is a particular faculty member that you may be interested in meeting. During your interviews be prompt, eager, and open to discuss your interests and application – ID providers tend to be detail oriented and quirky. Make sure you get to meet and speak earnestly with current fellows. Interviews should be followed up with thank yous and staying in touch with program directors and coordinators if strong interest is present.

Fellowship

Fellowship is a quick 3 years of training. Your experience can vary significantly based on the program style and hospital system you are in for training. The key components for a successful training are finding a mentor in the first year of training, being in open direct communication with your program director, and learning to balance clinical work with other interests over time.

Career Options

After fellowship, infectious diseases physicians have a variety of career options available depending on their interest and lifestyle. It is important throughout fellowship to talk with a mentor about career plans and options.

The most direct career path is clinical practice. This career is a needed service and there are many job postings each year. However, potential downsides can be availability of clinical careers at certain centers or locations and reimbursement for work. Infectious diseases is primarily a cerebral field, with limited options for procedures. It is consult and referral driven. Current payment structures can limit clinical compensation, or positions at a particular location. ID providers may do additional tasks to supplement income including research, time on committees, directing a subgroup such as ASP or infection prevention, or working as a hospitalist or clinic physician. This being noted, most ID providers have very high job satisfaction, longevity of practice, and enjoy flexibility of practice.

Research is the other major career path that many ID providers will pursue. These providers can focus on primarily performing research. Their niche may develop during fellowship, or after. If research is important to you, it is essential to learn and understand the nuances of grant writing and funding, as well as the art of negotiating for protected research time if you are also doing clinical practice. In addition to bench and translational research, clinical and quality improvement (QI) research are prominent in ID as well. If these areas are interesting to you, asking for additional training or support will be advantageous.

Key areas often not considered but in demand for ID physicians are careers in industry and regulatory branches. These two aspects are linked with clinical and research but are their own entities. People often will work for both sides at different times in their careers. Industry is important in making new drugs, treatments, and diagnostic products, and following them as they are researched, developed, and brought to market. They will fund research projects and push clinical boundaries. Financially, they tend to reimburse well for the work provided. Work, however, can be intermittent or based on social and economic determinants, and as an employee, you may encounter social or ethical quandaries that some may have difficulty addressing. The flipside of industry is regulation such as the Food and Drug Administration (FDA) or the US Department of Agriculture (USDA). These careers focus on regulation of industry and or clinical practice. The goals of focus are safety, efficacy, surveillance, and prevention, depending on the group. Careers tend to be stable, though may fluctuate depending on government funding. Working in regulation may be fulfilling for those not necessarily interested in clinical practice, although there may be some pressure from society and industry, who may feel hindered by regulatory bodies.

Other career options can focus on epidemiology, disaster relief, global health, and nonprofit groups. Many of these positions are difficult to find as they are not always well advertised. One sought-after position is becoming an Epidemic Intelligence Service (EIS) agent with the Centers for Disease Control (CDC). Private groups such as the Bill and Melinda Gates foundation provide opportunities that can be of interest for those with global health inclinations as well.

Helpful Resources

The Pediatric Infectious Diseases Society. https://www.pids.org
The Infectious Diseases Society of America https://www.IDsociety.org
Society for Healthcare Epidemiology of America https://www.shea-online.org
CDC Learning Connection https://www.cdc.gov/learning/index.html

Neonatal-Perinatal Medicine Fellowship

8

Sharla Rent, Dmitry Dukhovny, and Shweta Parmekar

Welcome to the exciting world of neonatology! A Neonatal-Perinatal Medicine (NPM) fellowship program will introduce you to the wide range of pathology, procedures, and personal connections that are integral to caring for newborns and their families. In this chapter we will introduce you to the key aspects of neonatology fellowship and life after training.

Choosing the Right Fellowship Program for You

The type of fellowship program you choose has a lot to do with the neonatal care you wish to practice after training. In practice, some neonatologists work in level IV neonatal intensive care units (NICUs) seeing the smallest and sickest newborns, while others work in regional NICUs with lower acuity. After fellowship, some physicians dedicate the bulk of their time to research,

S. Rent (✉)
Duke University, Durham, NC, USA
e-mail: Sharla.Rent@Duke.edu

D. Dukhovny
Oregon Health and Science University, Portland, OR, USA
e-mail: dukhovny@ohsu.edu

S. Parmekar
Baylor College of Medicine, Huston, TX, USA

57

while others focus their time on bedside care. After training, you will have the choice of working full time, part-time, or fulfilling clinical duties within the NICU as well as through other hospital roles. A NPM fellowship program must prepare their fellows for *any* of these future paths. Of course, training programs across the country are not identical, nor are their affiliated NICUs. When researching fellowship programs, ask yourself the following questions:

- What am I passionate about? What are my research interests?
- Is there a potential mentor at the institution that I am excited to work with?
- What lifestyle do I ultimately want? Do I see myself working in a primary clinical role or a research role or an administrative role?
- Are there other factors, such as a significant other or kids, or personal interests, which I should factor in to my decision making (e.g., should geographical location be considered based on partner's work, family)?

Not everyone will know the answers to these questions before starting – and that's okay! Most people won't know what they want their faculty role to look like before starting fellowship. The key point is to spend time thinking about what is important to you and if the centers you are looking at will meet those needs. Fellowship programs allow you to tailor your research time to your academic interests, so investing time from the start to reflect on what those interests are is important. Consider the examples below (Fig. 8.1) about how you may translate an interest into opportunities available at a program.

Finding the Right Research Project and Mentor

Research, or scholarly activity, during fellowship is one of the most unique and exciting aspects of subspecialty training in pediatrics. Depending on the fellowship program, at least half of your

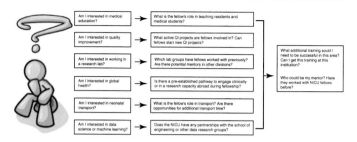

Fig. 8.1 Translating personal interest into scholarly work

3 years is devoted to scholarly activity. For some, scholarly activity during NPM fellowship is an extension of their prior work (e.g., PhD or Masters). For others, this might be their first exposure to dedicated research time during their career. Regardless of your past research experience, having a good mentor throughout your NPM fellowship is important.

There is no one best approach to identifying a research mentor, but there are a few steps everyone can and should follow at the start:

1. Explore your interests with your program leadership – either your fellowship director or designated faculty is assigned to help fellows start the exploration.
2. Think about what you want to do and what are some of the strengths at your institution.
   - If you don't know where to start, consider which broad areas of scholarship most interests you: basic and translational science, clinical research, health services and epidemiologic research, medical education, or quality improvement and patient safety.
3. Talk to the faculty within your division.
   - Capitalize on the informal opportunities while on service to find out what faculty members do with their nonclinical time and how their careers have evolved over time; for more junior faculty, ask about their fellowship research experiences.

4. Explore mentors outside of your divisions.
   • Almost all NPM fellowships are based at large academic centers or have an affiliation with one. If there is someone outside of the division or department who does something that overlaps your interest, set up a meeting with them.
5. Think about how your scholarly activity may align with your next career steps as a junior attending. This is a great time to explore something new or build on your current portfolio.

Your fellowship project does not have to be the beginning of your career's work. Instead you can think of it as a stepping stone, where you are building skills to add to your scholarship toolbox. Ultimately, no matter what your next career move is, scholarly activity during fellowship will help you become a better clinician by learning to ask the right questions, incorporating current evidence, thinking outside of the box, and better advocating for your patient and their families.

Choosing the right mentor is a key to your success. The faculty and program leadership in your fellowship will help you identify mentors based on experience of previous fellows and junior faculty. Make sure that they are ready to take you on as a mentee and that they have the time to do so. What you, as a fellow, are providing is time, interest, and dedication. In return, you should get mentorship and support. Explore and meet with lots of different people. Setting a meeting is not a commitment – think of it as speed dating. You never know who you may meet and what opportunities may come from it later.

Lastly, although neonatology is the largest pediatric subspecialty, the field is still relatively small and global. There may be opportunities to expand your mentorship network through long-distance mentoring. It's a great opportunity to explore, although you must always have someone locally as well to ensure you get proper support and continue your progress.

Networking on a National Scale

There are approximately 250 fellows entering NPM fellowship each year and over 5000 neonatologists in the USA. There are many opportunities to expand your network, starting within your own hospital/division. Most states now have a perinatal quality collaborative (PQC), either in a formal structure or informal gathering of the local NICUs. The work of state PQCs probably has the biggest impact on the public health for your region when it comes to perinatal services, plus it's an opportunity to meet and collaborate with colleagues with whom you may exchange patients and frequently talk on the phone or telemedicine.

The largest organization of neonatologists is through the American Academy of Pediatrics (AAP) Section of Neonatal Perinatal Medicine (SONPM). Within that organization, you will find a home for everyone, no matter the stage of your career. Most relevant to the fellows and junior attendings is the Trainee and Early Career Neonatologist (TECaN) subgroup of the section, which was founded circa 2008 and has tremendously grown the resources to help ensure success and transition of fellows and junior neonatologists (Fig. 8.2).

In addition, the AAP is the largest advocate for all pediatrics in the local, regional, and federal governments; thus being an active and supportive member of the AAP is a statement of public health support and advocacy for all children and families. In addition to the national SoNPM, your AAP state chapter may be a great resource and home for local advocacy.

Within the AAP, there are other sections that may align with your interests – whether it's global health or advocacy, you can find additional resources and networks. There are many other organizations in addition to the AAP that may be of interest to you. Often, these organizations align with clinical, research, or

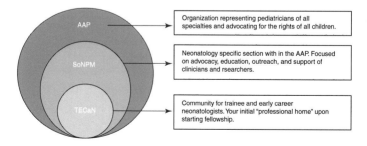

Fig. 8.2 Relationship between AAP, SoNPM, and TECaN

administrative interests. For example, if quality improvement and patient safety is your area of focus, then the Vermont Oxford Network (VON) is the perfect hodgepodge of networking with US and world experts in quality improvement. The VON Annual Quality Congress is one of the few meetings that is truly multidisciplinary and includes the family voice. In addition to the local work (because all improvement starts local!), VON has tremendously grown their global health network over the recent years. Talk to your faculty and research mentors, and explore the different opportunities that align with your interests.

Planning a Career in Neonatology

You may have come into the fellowship knowing exactly what your future career would entail or you may have embarked on a journey to discover your options throughout training. As you near the end of your training, reflect on which type of patients you enjoyed caring for the most and if you had the opportunity to train in several facilities, which type of unit do you gravitate to. Some attending positions will place you primarily within a single unit, while others may require you to cover multiple hospitals. Some units have dedicated NICU respiratory therapists, nurse practitioners, access to medical and surgical subspecialists, and frequently use technologies such as extracorporeal membrane oxygenation (ECMO). Other units are unable to admit high-risk infants below a particular gestational age or support those requiring significant respiratory support, necessitating transfer of these infants to a higher-level NICU. Consider the neonatal population you enjoy caring for the most and what type of physician role you will find the most fulfilling.

Beyond the unit structure, there are several important aspects of your role to consider:

- Will you be working with medical students, trainees, or advanced practitioners? What will your role be in terms of training and supervision?
- What is the patient to provider ratio?

- Who attends deliveries?
- What is the call frequency? Do attendings stay in the hospital overnight ("in-house call") or do they take call from home?

The relative importance of each aspect of your future role will vary person to person, and it is important to use your time in fellowship to figure out what is most important to you in your career and life. As you negotiate your job, the salary is just one aspect of it. The aforementioned clinical factors in addition to the academic/nonclinical support provided are just as critical to consider when it comes to job satisfaction and work life integration.

But First…Boards

The NPM boards are typically offered every other year. As a new attending, it is important to plan ahead and ensure that you have enough time to adequately prepare for this exam. Most academic centers and practices will accommodate this need within your clinical schedule. Exam registration fees will cost you approximately $3000 and are typically due several months before the exam, so have this amount set aside or better yet discuss these costs during contract negotiations. Institutional or practice compensation for the initial certifying board exam and board preparatory courses vary widely.

It is essential that you have a game plan for studying. Even if you have diligently read neonatology textbooks cover to cover, completed all the Prep questions, and read all the NeoReviews articles, a successful performance on the board exam requires detailed attention to the high-yield content areas that you may not have considered or spent an inordinate amount of time reviewing. It may be helpful to use the American Board of Pediatrics (ABP) Neonatal-Perinatal Content Specifications Outline as a guide to identify content areas you may need to focus on.

The nuances of when to start studying, what materials to use, and whose advice to listen to are largely dependent on you. You have taken and passed multiple board examinations to reach this stage and already have some idea of what works best for you. What has worked for others may not be the best for your schedule, budget, or simply how you learn best. Spend some time thinking about how much time you'll need or have, how much money you are willing to spend, and what books and question materials you'd like to use.

One approach to board preparation is to attend one of the several comprehensive, intensive review courses offered annually at varying US cities that encompass physiology and pathophysiology of high-yield neonatal perinatal medicine. Keep in mind these usually come with a price tag of $2000–$3000 after registration, travel, lodging, etc. If you are unable to attend one of these courses for any reason, then you are not alone. Plenty of board takers choose self-study as an alternative to these courses to meet their needs. Create accountability for yourself with a timeline of content material, readings, questions, and images you'd like to review. Be honest with yourself about how much time you'll need for this and leave cushion for those areas that may give you some trouble. The bottom line is with a little bit of planning you can successfully fulfill your commitments and prepare for and pass your boards.

Pediatric Palliative Care Fellowship

Jaime Jump

Application Process

Pediatric hospice and palliative medicine fellowship is a 1-year fellowship training program available to candidates who have completed an Accreditation Council for Graduate Medical Education (ACGME-Allopathic) or American Osteopathic Association (AOA-osteopathic) accredited program in child neurology, family medicine, internal medicine, pediatrics, physical medicine and rehabilitation, or neurology. Other eligible candidates include those with at least three clinical years in an ACGME- or AOA-accredited GME program in one of the following specialties: anesthesiology, emergency medicine, obstetrics and gynecology, psychiatry, radiation oncology, radiology, or surgery. Pediatric hospice and palliative medicine fellowship is unique in that it is not exclusive to primary pediatric-trained physicians. As of the writing of this chapter, there are 36 ACGME-accredited training programs/pediatric tracks, which offer one to two fellowship positions per program each year.

J. Jump (✉)
Baylor College of Medicine, Houston, TX, USA

Sections of Critical Care and Palliative Care, Texas Children's Hospital, Houston, TX, USA
e-mail: jxjump@texaschildrens.org

© The Author(s), under exclusive license to Springer Nature Switzerland AG 2021
P. M. Garrett, K. Yoon-Flannery (eds.), *A Pediatrician's Path*,
https://doi.org/10.1007/978-3-030-75370-2_9

65

To begin your application, you will need to register with both Electronic Residency Application Service (ERAS) and the National Resident Matching Program (NRMP) to be eligible for the match. Both ERAS and NRMP publish instructions and a timeline for application on their respective websites each year. Candidates apply in the summer prior to the start date of their prospective fellowship. Pediatric hospice and palliative medicine fellowship is unique because the match occurs under the realm of the National Resident Matching Program (NRMP) or Medical Specialties Matching Program (MSMP) and not under the Pediatric Subspecialty Match. ERAS will prompt the submission of required documents including at least three letters of reference. After the application is complete, interview offers will either be made via e-mail or within the ERAS system that automatically includes program-specific interview dates. Interviews generally extend from August to early November.

The key to a successful match is an early application submission. Many successful candidates have their application nearly complete by the time NRMP opens. It is important to research programs during this time and mentally prioritize the programs that tailor to your specific fellowship interests. Remember that strong recommendation letters are often obtained from mentors who know you well not only as a physician but also as a person. Seek these letters out as early as possible as a professional courtesy to allow adequate time for the writer to complete it. Seek out opportunities to practice your interview skills and to prepare for possible questions. Most importantly, be yourself. Hospice and palliative medicine fellowships highly value your interpersonal relatability and your ability to work within a large interdisciplinary team. If you are approaching the end of the interview season and have not received an interview invite from a program that has been high on your list, consider sending an e-mail directly to the program director asking for possible reconsideration of your application. You may not receive a response to this request or the response may not be what you would have hoped for, but it is definitely worth a shot. Make sure to send thank you notes after you complete the interview process with a prospective program. Snail mail thank you notes are preferred, but e-mail will suffice if you are running low on time. Thank you notes may seem like a small gesture, but they really help you stand out during the process and highlights your interest in the prospective program.

After the interview season is complete, rank lists will be due in the NRMP system a little less than 1 month before match day. It is important to be thoughtful about your rank list and consider only ranking programs where you feel you will be a good fit. This will contribute greatly to your success during training as a hospice and palliative medicine fellow. It is to be noted that this fellowship is an extremely emotionally demanding year given the nature of the subspecialty and the large amount of continuous clinical service condensed into a short 1-year fellowship training.

You will be notified via e-mail by the NRMP on Match Day with your match results. NRMP will also publish the match results listed by each training program. If you fail to match, the NRMP will provide a list of programs that went unmatched. In this circumstance, it would be wise to seek advice about proceeding with an application to an unmatched program or potentially waiting another year to apply with the next cycle. The most updated list of available pediatric hospice and palliative medicine fellowships and tracks can be found here: http://aahpm.org/uploads/Pediatric_Palliative_Care_Fellowships_and_Pediatric_Tracks_Update_12.18.19.pdf

Fellowship Training

Comprehensive core competencies for training hospice and palliative medicine physicians have been developed by a Hospice and Palliative Medicine Project Work Group and can be found here:

http://aahpm.org/uploads/education/competencies/
Competencies%20v.%202.3.pdf.

Although no hospice and palliative medicine fellowship curriculum is exactly the same, the goal of this fellowship is to become competent in providing palliative care consultation in the inpatient and outpatient setting and to understand the management of hospice patients. Since pediatric hospice and palliative medicine fellowship is a short 1-year fellowship, you can expect the majority of your time to be spent performing clinical patient care with dedicated time to design and implement a small scholarly project usually related to quality improvement, research, or education.

Hospice and palliative medicine fellowship curricula will vary based on the individual program. Core rotations can have some variation based on individual institution resources but usually includes inpatient palliative care consults, home hospice and outpatient palliative care consults, long-term care or complex care service, hospice, dedicated scholarly project time, and electives that can range from radiation oncology to maternal fetal medicine.

Another unique feature to hospice and palliative medicine fellowship is that although the subspecialty is recognized by the American Board of Pediatrics (ABP), the board examination falls under the realm of the American Board of Internal Medicine, and all trainees in hospice and palliative medicine (both adult and pediatric) take the same board examination. Fellowship didactics will be centered around core topics in palliative care including advanced symptom management, end-of-life care, and complex care coordination and communication. The didactic sessions also typically include adjunct learning related to adult hospice and palliative medicine topics that will be addressed on the board examination.

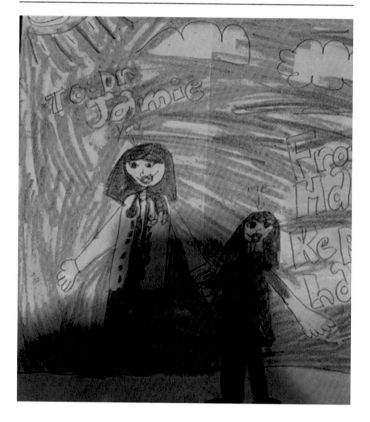

What to Look for in a Program

The pediatric palliative care community is a small, close-knit community that networks well across many forums, most notably the Annual Assembly of the American Academy of Hospice and Palliative Medicine (AAHPM). I recommend attending the annual assembly, if possible, the year prior to applying for fellowship.

The assembly will allow you to network within the community and to get a feel for the interests and expertise of many of the faculty that are very involved with training pediatric hospice and palliative medicine fellows. As with all fellowship programs, each program varies in size, scope of practice, and opportunities. The majority of postgraduate hospice and palliative medicine fellows will consider a job in either an academic program or a community-based hospital program. Although it is not mandatory that you have an exact plan as to how you would like to use your hospice and palliative medicine training, it is often helpful to have some insight into what you think will be your passions within the field so that you can focus your fellowship search appropriately.

It is to be noted that any pediatric hospice and palliative medicine fellowship is both academically and emotionally demanding. Your personal fit within a program is important to your academic and emotional growth and your ability to perform good self-care during this training year. Hospice and palliative medicine is a team sport, and it is important that you feel comfortable being vulnerable and adaptable with all members of the interdisciplinary team.

Lifestyle

As a pediatric hospice and palliative medicine fellow, your hours will vary depending on your rotation and the demands of your inpatient or outpatient service. Some of your days can be a more predictable 9 am to 5 pm hours; however, many days, the needs of patients and families including tasks like family meetings can be variable and unpredictable. Flexibility is going to be key to your learning because you are not only available while in the hospital setting but will likely be on call while on service to discuss symptom management and in some programs, to manage outpatient hospice patients in the community.

Beyond the hard work, expect to have fun! You will be part of a large interdisciplinary team that likes to share lunches, life events, laughs, and tears. The year will be extremely challenging and rewarding. Remember to be genuine and to be yourself because that is who both your team and your families will trust.

Post Pediatric Portal Program

10

Gabriela Andrade

Introduction

What is the Post Pediatric Portal Program (PPPP) and why is it in the fellowship section of this book? The truth is that this is not a well-known training track because it is relatively new, but a gem of a physician career path. In this chapter we will discuss what this program entails, if it is right for you, and the career opportunities this training will open for you.

The Basics

The PPPP was created in 2007 in response to the severe shortage in child and adolescent psychiatrists in the United States [1]. The American Board of Psychiatry and Neurology (ABPN) approved a program that allows for any board eligible pediatrician to complete a 36-month training experience that meets the requirements for board certification in both general psychiatry and child/adolescent psychiatry. This means that you will be eligible to be triple boarded in pediatrics, adult psychiatry, and child psychiatry at the completion of this training.

G. Andrade (✉)
The Children's Hospital of Philadelphia, Philadelphia, PA, USA

P. M. Garrett, K. Yoon-Flannery (eds.), *A Pediatrician's Path*,
https://doi.org/10.1007/978-3-030-75370-2_10

Applicants

PPPP applicants must have completed an ACGME accredited pediatric residency [2]. Outside of this requirement, applicants come from varied backgrounds. There is a mix of physicians that have recently completed their pediatric residency and want to go straight into this subspeciality area, while others are mid- to later career pediatricians that want to go back to augment their skill set or make a change in their career. This diverse applicant pool makes this program both competitive and accessible to all pediatricians no matter where they are in their career.

Programs

As of early 2021, there are four training sites which offer this program:

- Case Western Reserve Hospital
- The Children's Hospital of Philadelphia
- University of Tennessee Health Science Center
- Medical College of Georgia

Each training program takes two fellows per year. Given the small community, something you will notice quickly is that all the program directors know each other well and really want to help you find the best program for your individual needs. I encourage anyone that is interested in this path to reach out to each program coordinator to become familiar with each program and learn what would work best for you. While the start date of the program is typically July first, applications are reviewed on an ongoing basis.

Breakdown of the Program

Though all programs have some slight difference in distribution of clinical rotations, all PPPP fellows will complete 18 months in General Psychiatry and 18 months in Child and Adolescent

Psychiatry (CAP). This means that all fellows will be doing rotations at the same ACGME-approved sites as the adult residents and CAP fellows.

Rotations will include but are not limited to:

- Addiction psychiatry
- Pediatric neurology
- Adult neurology
- Geriatric psychiatry
- Inpatient child and adolescent psychiatry
- Inpatient general psychiatry
- Adult outpatient psychiatry
- Child and adolescent outpatient psychiatry
- Child and adolescent consult liaison psychiatry
- Adult consult liaison psychiatry
- Emergency psychiatry
- Forensic psychiatry

Job Opportunities

The job opportunities and lifestyle options for PPPP graduates are excellent. Many surveys have shown that child and adolescent psychiatrists rank the first or second of all medical specialties in the average number of job offers per trainee after graduation [3]. After completing the PPPP, you will not only meet those qualifications but you will also have your pediatrics training to bolster your resume even further.

Since there is such a great demand for child and adolescent psychiatrists, graduates also fare extremely well when it comes to the diversity of practice options, lifestyle, and job flexibility. Graduates of Post Pediatric Portal Program can choose to work in a variety of settings including:

- Integrated mental healthcare
- Primary care settings
- Outpatient academic psychiatry
- Private general psychiatry
- Outpatient academic or private child and adolescent psychiatry

- Consultation-liaison
- Emergency psychiatry

Some choose to continue to practice all three specialties (pediatrics, adult psychiatry, and child psychiatry) individually, while others decide to dedicate themselves to one area or fuse their training to meet a specific need. Your choices truly are endless!

References

1. Pilot program trains pediatricians in child and adolescent psychiatry. Robert Ellis and Amy Kathryn Anderson. AAP News November 2010;31(11):31. https://doi.org/10.1542/aapnews.20103111-31.
2. https://tripleboard-postpediatricportal.com/.
3. https://www.aacap.org/aacap/Medical_Students_and_Residents/Residents_and_Fellows/Child_and_Adolescent_Psychiatry_as_a_Career.aspx.

Completion of Multiple Fellowships: Finding a Job

Jaime Jump

Introduction

I found over the course of my very long training (I will share part of my story later in this chapter) that the climate surrounding medical training has changed. More often than not, I found that I was surrounded by more and more colleagues who were also pursuing fellowships (sometimes multiple) after completing their residency training. It is hard to pinpoint exactly when or why the culture shifted from primary care to subspecialty care, but it is a real phenomenon. In this chapter, I hope to share some of my experience and challenges with the job search as a multiple subspecialty trained physician. Looking back, I wish I did not head into the job search so naïve to the realities of practicing in multiple subspecialties.

As a caveat, I could have never predicted writing this chapter during the very challenging and unknown time of the COVID-19 pandemic. Right now, the entire world, especially frontline healthcare workers, are living in a time of unprecedented change. Social distancing, employee screening and changes in practice and salary cuts, all never before a worry for physicians, have become a daily source of anxiety. My hope for all of you taking the time to

J. Jump (✉)
Baylor College of Medicine, Houston, TX, USA

Sections of Critical Care and Palliative Care, Texas Children's Hospital, Houston, TX, USA
e-mail: jxjump@texaschildrens.org

read this chapter is that the above topics are irrelevant and that you can pursue your passions without the worries and limitations of a worldwide health crisis.

My Story

As I mentioned earlier, I took the long road to my end goal career as both pediatric critical care and pediatric palliative care physician. The responses I hear from physician colleagues after telling them what I practice is usually twofold. The first response is usually something along the lines of being crazy, sad/depressed, or an adrenaline junkie. The second response is very different and goes something like, "Awesome! You should be so marketable. The job search should be a slam dunk for you!" Although I cannot pretend that we are not our own kind of crazy and that I am not a little bit of an adrenaline junkie, I was also falsely reassured that my job search would be an easy one after 11 years of being a student and trainee. Unfortunately, it turned out that my assumptions were very wrong.

I went through the job search process receiving multiple emails back from programs that were interested in what I had to offer. However, after one or two interviews, I began to feel like I was going to have to give up some part of my hard-earned training and skills to find a suitable job. I had trained in two subspecialties that seemed to go hand in hand, but for some programs, it was not seen that way. I tackled the extremes of being offered full-time critical care positions with the expectations of creating a new palliative care program in my administrative time (not possible) to giving up formal palliative care practice for a full-time critical care position. The process was overwhelming and, on some days, extremely devastating considering all of my hard work and dedication to both fields. At the end of the day, I interviewed at only two academic programs who were interested in supporting both my critical care and palliative care careers. However, there was some risk in only interviewing at two instutions that I felt were a good fit to support my career goals. I wasn't guaranteed a job offer at either of these institutions, and if I was, they were both outside of my geographic comfort zone and would require a cross-country move. The good news is that I ended up getting an offer at one of these institutions and I'm now a native Northeasterner thriving as a Texan. The bottom line is if you are graduating with multi-subspecialty training under your belt, be open-minded and, if possible, unrestricted geographically. The rest of this chapter will focus on the academic job search pearls for the multi-subspecialty-trained physician.

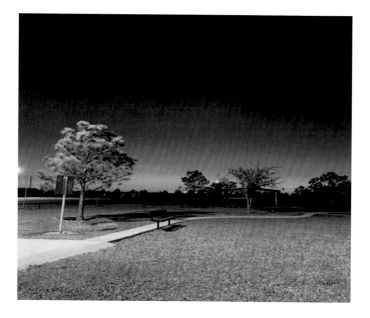

Start Early

I would recommend starting to scour the job listings in October and November during your last year of training. It is nice to get a feel for what is being posted and what types of jobs may pique your interest. Once you find these types of jobs, do your homework. Do some reading about the institution and the faculty and use your resources. By the time you are at the end of your training, many of your friends and colleagues from residency and fellowship may already be working in their respective field in institutions across the country. Reach out to them and ask them questions about their current jobs. Don't be afraid to reach out to institutions of interest even if their jobs are not posted on the typical job search websites for each subspecialty. This occurs quite often, and it is often worth sending an email to the section chiefs of your subspecialties at that institution to inquire about possible job opportunities.

The goal of starting early is to be able to narrow down a list of places to start sending out emails that show your interest in available positions. These emails should ideally include a cover letter and an updated CV. Therefore, the early search should motivate you not to procrastinate completing these items. Once you send out some emails that express your interest in the respective positions, the responses will be varied. Some institutions will require you to submit these emails to a recruiter that will act as a liaison between you and the section chief to determine if you are a good fit for an interview invite. Other institutions may have you in direct contact with the chief of the sections. The timeline for interviews can start as early as November and usually concludes around mid- to late February. Contract offers and negotiations usually occur and are completed by March or April for start dates in the upcoming academic year, usually July or later.

Geography

Geography is a tough topic to give advice about because most of the decisions surrounding the "where" of getting a job are personal. You may have a spouse that needs to stay in a geographic area for work or older children that are comfortable in their current schools and activities. That being said, if you are in a situation that allows you to explore jobs outside of your geographic comfort zone, do it! Job availability differs vastly one year to the next based on hospital expansions, patient volumes, and a multitude of other factors that are above our pay grade. Frankly, a large percentage of where you find job openings in your subspecialty may be luck of the draw.

Geographic exploration can also be a reason to start the job search early. If you have a significant other, start the conversation about locations you'd be willing to try out a new zip code. If you are offered an interview in an area that you know nothing about but it seems to fit your personal and professional needs, go check it out. If your schedule allows, plan some extra days surrounding your interview days to allow time to explore the area. Many times, academic institutions will have a two-step interview process that will allow you to visit the city multiple times. Sometimes, during the second interview, the institution may offer to cover travel expenses for your significant other so that you can both explore the area. It is also common to be offered a community tour with a realtor that can give you a feel for housing opportunities and affordability.

Final Thoughts

Remember your worth as a multiple subspecialty-trained physician. You are rare and extremely valuable to any institution where you decide to work. Don't settle for good enough if there is an opportunity that will allow you to jumpstart your career the way you always planned. When you finally sign your first job contract, you may have some anxiety about the feeling of finality associated with that commitment. I think it's very important to keep the decision in perspective and know that often, most people don't stay in their first job for more than 1 to 3 years. If the job ends up not being a good fit, learn as much as you can and seek out another opportunity that will allow you to pursue your clinical and academic interests in a way that you will find fulfilling.

Part II

Your First Job Search

Your First Job: Where to Look

12

Namrita Odackal

You've trained for years, been on call for countless nights, sacrificed so many holidays and friends' weddings – all so you could get to this point, finding your first job as an attending physician. While this is the anticipated beginning of the rest of our lives for so many of us, be aware that this is a lot of pressure to put on yourself. Finding your first job out of residency or fellowship can be a long humbling process that tests your patience. This can be a lot about being in the right place at the right time, or even knowing the right person. Flexibility will be your friend. Approach this process with an open mind. Find comfort in the fact that your first job does not have to be your dream job. And know that polite persistence is key.

Looking for a Job

When to Start Looking

When to start looking depends a lot on how much thought you have already given this process. Your approach will be very different if you have spent years knowing exactly where you

N. Odackal (✉)
Neonatology, North Denver Envision Group, Louisville, CO, USA

want to work, and nothing else will do – than if you still haven't decided if you want an academic career or are more interested in private practice. It also doesn't have to necessarily be either-or.

The first step is to try to prioritize what is important to you in your career. Be able to answer – "Where do I want to be in 5 years…in 10 years…in 20 years?" – and be comfortable with that answer. Be honest with yourself. You may be interested in a 70% research/30% clinical position, you might be enthusiastic about teaching trainees, you might want to finally reacquaint yourself with the artist in you and pursue a part-time position that affords you more flexibility, or you may be primarily driven by a geographic location that brings you close to family. Once you have your priorities straight, and know what you can bend on and what is a deal-breaker – your job search will be easier to organize.

If you are interested in a heavily research-focused position, you should start thinking about your future job soon after you begin your last phase of training, whether that is a residency or a fellowship. Give yourself time to pursue and demonstrate particular accomplishments, i.e., publications or grants, which some positions may expect of you. If you dream of being a Program Director or an assistant Program Director eventually, consider the role of chief resident or chief fellow. Explore potential supplemental degrees in medical education. If you are interested in global health and want a position that provides you time to travel for Helping Babies Breathe, for instance, you should explore these opportunities during training. Cue yourself up for success by demonstrating enthusiasm and that skill set within your training program.

You should seriously begin the search for jobs in the spring prior to the last year of your training. This gives you ample time to explore different geographic locations, familiarize yourself with the resources available, and communicate with the people who will help you along this process without stressing either them or you out.

Where to Look

People

There are likely several resources available to you through your training program. Frequently, your *Program Director* and other *mentors* have helpful contacts within your institution, your region, or your specific field that may know of job opportunities or have connections with people who may know of them. These will be people who you have worked with in training, who can vouch for you, and generally who feel invested in your success. Set up meetings with them, discuss your priorities, and follow up on the leads they provide.

Contact the *graduated trainees* in the years above you as well. They went through this process not long ago and may be at an institution you want to go to, have recommendations for or against certain jobs based on their experience, and be able to provide you other helpful tips. If you have *peers you met at conferences*, frequently they may have insider information on what positions could be available in their regions. If you have made contacts with any program directors or medical directors during conferences, now is the time to reach out to them and express your interest. Make use of all the networking you've done over the past several years.

If you are looking for private positions, there are usually *recruiters* who are the best point person to contact. For example, Mednax and Envision have regional recruiters who can help you navigate and apply to available positions within your interest. Once you contact them, they will communicate with you when relevant positions become available and coordinate interviews. The same goes for locum positions – you can contact the company (e.g., CompHealth, Weatherby, LocumTenens) and they will connect with you an *agent* who will become your main contact for positions that are of interest to you.

Although not common, you may choose to hire a *headhunter*. Headhunters will actively try to find a position for you but will likely charge you a fee for this service.

Websites

The websites available for physician job searches are of variable quality. I will list a few here that are commonly used. If you are applying for a subspecialty position, there may be specific websites that are more helpful; ask fellows you know that have gone through the process. Be wary of posting your CV on a lot of these websites – frequently once you do, you will be inundated with phone calls from a variety of companies who most likely will just be wasting your time. Instead, apply specifically to positions that appeal to you, ideally with a cover letter and CV (see more on *applications* later). You can set up alerts at many of these websites so that they contact you once a position becomes available that matches your search criteria. Some general job search websites include Monster.com and Ziprecruiter.com. Job search websites specific to physicians include CareerMD.com, PraticeLink.com, NEJMcareercenter.org, Mednax.com, and jobs.pedjobs.org.

Networking Opportunities

There are both in-person and online career fairs geared toward individuals like you who are job-searching. The American Academy of Pediatrics holds virtual career fairs every few months. Get on their career center Listserv to be contacted about these. You can communicate with recruiters from many regions and institutions during these online sessions. If you have the chance to attend a conference during training in your second or third year, turn it into an opportunity to network and meet senior members from institutions you may want to work with. Recruiters are present at many of these conferences as well. Make use of this time to make connections that you can call on during your job search.

Your First Job: Applications and Interviews

13

Namrita Odackal

Now that you have explored job opportunities, it is time to think about your application and interviews.

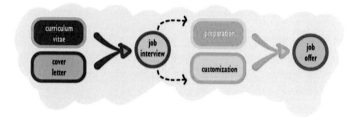

Application

Your application for a job position will primarily consist of two things, your CV and a cover letter. You can begin your application for jobs prior to even finding one that you are interested in!

N. Odackal (✉)
Neonatology, North Denver Envision Group, Louisville, CO, USA

Curriculum Vitae

Chances are you have a preliminary version of your curriculum vitae (CV) ready to go already. If not, start it now and keep it updated as you proceed through training. Ask for examples of CVs from your peers, and keep a collection of the CVs you may come across during your training to work off of for formatting. Generally, do not include accomplishments prior to medical school. Have three references at the end of your CV (and make sure they know you are using them as a reference) whom you believe will be strong advocates of your application. Including a Medical Director, Program Director, or Division Chief makes a strong impression. Make sure to have your final CV proofread by mentors who have ample experience looking at CVs and hiring physicians.

You may even want to have a few different variations of your CV prepared depending on which type of job you are submitting it for. A CV for an academic position may focus especially on teaching experience, while one for a private community practice may focus more on quality improvement work. Whenever you write an email to express interest in a position, make sure to attach your CV. If you have an update to your CV during the application process (i.e., a new publication), use the opportunity to send an updated CV as a great excuse to touch base again with your contact for that position.

Cover Letter

You should also have a base cover letter prepared, which you should ideally modify and customize for each position you are applying for. Cover letters should be no more than a page long. Include why you are interested in the specific position, what makes you stand out as an applicant, and what you will be able to contribute if they were to choose you. Ideally, the reader should come away with a better understanding of who you are as an applicant than if they had just read your CV.

Depending on what your initial form of contact is for the position, you may or may not want to include the cover letter from the beginning. If you are "cold calling" just to see if a position is open, don't include the cover letter – just attach your CV. If you are officially applying to a position from a website, then include both your CV and the cover letter.

Interview Process

If you receive an invite for an interview, that is half the battle! Be prepared to interview as soon as you apply. Practice with mentors beforehand. The first contact the point person may have with you could be a phone call which serves as a behavioral interview, or it could be an email requesting to set up a time for you to meet in person. The point person could be a recruiter or the division head! You have to be ready for either because it will be your first impression and it could be your last.

Have answers ready to go for all the basic interview questions you have ever heard of such as "tell me about yourself?," "what is your ideal job?," "where do you see yourself in 5 years?," "why do you want to apply here?," and "what are your strengths and weaknesses." Be prepared to speak intelligently about anything on your CV and practice weaving in details about yourself that you think are important into conversation. Make sure you have researched their unit and looked at resources from their website and have questions ready for them that show you have been thoughtful about the information that is available to you. If possible, mention specific individuals within the program that you would like to meet with. If you are interested in a particular research topic, have people in mind that might serve as mentors and have looked into their research already.

Depending on the position, you may have a series of phone calls or online meetings before actually meeting your future colleagues in person. Typically, for job interviews, the hospital or practice will take on the expenses for your travel and lodging during the interview, so they want to know you are serious before investing the resources. You will need to arrange time away from your training in order to pursue your interviews so make sure to plan accordingly.

Before an interview, you will usually receive a list of the people you will be meeting and instructions on where to park, where to go, etc. Ideally, you should have specific questions for the different individuals, although feel free to repeat some of the questions to get different perspectives. Remember, you are evaluating them as well to see if you and the job are a good match. Interviews for academic positions may ask you to do a presentation on your research or other accomplishments. Make sure to practice this ahead of time with a critical audience. Of course, be as professional as possible – show up early, wear a suit, be as well rested as your schedule allows. Bring a copy of your CV and, if applicable, research with you, in case it comes up. Bring something to take notes on. After your interview, make sure to write down your thoughts. Follow up with the individuals you interviewed with to thank them for their time, to express your interest, and to find out next steps.

Contract Considerations: Negotiating the Contract

14

Joannie Yeh

Overview

Contract negotiation is an important step in the journey to searching for the right job after residency. While you may be attracted to an ideal job description, *staying* attracted to that job after you start working there depends on how you negotiate the details in your contract. This process requires preparation of both mindset and data. Medical school tuition and residency training salary leave little room for negotiation, so a shift in mindset is required to realize that everything is negotiable. In order to have successful asks, data are required to guide how and what you bring to the negotiation table. This chapter will take you through a few steps to understand and prepare for this process.

The Ask Mindset

Throughout medical training, we do what we are told and we accept what we are given. There is no negotiating work hours. There is no negotiating medical school tuition or residency salary.

J. Yeh (✉)
Sidney Kimmel Medical College, Philadelphia, PA, USA

P. M. Garrett, K. Yoon-Flannery (eds.), *A Pediatrician's Path*,
https://doi.org/10.1007/978-3-030-75370-2_14

With a job, however, we can ask for things. We do not have to accept the job offer as is. In fact, we shouldn't. We should ask for more – more administrative time, more vacation time, more continuing medical education money, more sign on bonus, more compensation.

Asking is normal.

Asking is expected.

Asking is what you deserve.

Here are a couple ways to get more comfortable with asking. Start by practicing with small things. Ask for extras when ordering food or coffee. Or ask for a side to be switched out for something that is more fitting to your taste. Ask for your cable or security system bill to be lowered. Ask a store employee to look in the back for more inventory if you can't find what you want. If something could be made better for you, ask for it. It's okay if someone says "no," but it is good practice to advocate for yourself, and eventually, someone will say "yes."

Now, think about how a description in a job posting could be made even better for you. Maybe the job setting is what you want, but the commute is long, so you would like longer and fewer shifts. Maybe the job requires working in several offices, but you only want to work in one or two. Maybe the job relies heavily on referrals, so you want the office marketing team to be flexible and available to you. Get in the practice of imagining not just how you fit into the job but also how the job could be made to better fit you.

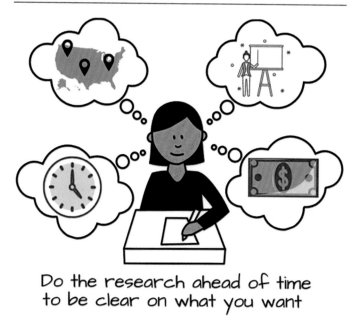

Do the research ahead of time
to be clear on what you want

What Do You Want and Need? What Do You *Not* Want?

Now that you realize that you are allowed to imagine the possibilities and to ask for them, it's time to map out what you want, what you need, and what you don't want in a job. Consider the following aspects of a job – location, roles, hours, required support staff and equipment, and opportunities for growth and promotion.

Roles: Do you want to teach? Ask for protected time to teach. Do you want to do research? Ask for protected time to write grants and publications. Do you want to only see a subset of patients? Ask for protected time to just see those patients.

Staff and equipment: Do you need certain staff to be efficient in seeing patients? Do you need a scribe? Do you want a certain number of patient rooms? Do you want a certain number of operating or procedure rooms? Is the current equipment sufficient for your procedures, and if not, is there a plan to purchase it and how will the cost be distributed?

Location: Do you want to work in a rural, suburban, or urban practice? How far are you willing to travel for your commute? Do you want to live in a rural, suburban, or urban community?

Hours: Do you have a limit to how much call you are willing to take? Is there flexibility to how long and which shifts you work? How many vacation and continuing education days do you want?

Career opportunities: Do you want an opportunity to become a practice owner? Do you want on-site grand rounds and other continuing medical education events? Does the organization have medical education or administrative positions that you might be interested in applying for now or in the future?

Practice type: Do you want to work in a hospital or an office? Do you want to work where the doctors are owners or where the practice is managed by a large organization? Do you want to start your own practice? How about less common paths like direct primary care or locum tenens?

How Much Do Other People in This Position Make?

We are a few pages into this chapter on contract negotiation, and we haven't even started to talk about money. That's because there is so much more to contract negotiations than just money. Without the ask mindset and the careful consideration of what you want to ask for, no amount of money will make the job fulfilling. When you understand what you want and need in order to do your job well and to have joy in it, asking for the money to do this job is a piece of cake. Here are some ways to find out how much to ask for.

The Medical Group Management Association (MGMA) has been keeping track of salaries and relative value units (RVUs – a measure of productivity) for physicians and all types of practice employees. It relies on surveys filled out by practice administrators for their data. They are available at a high price, but the information is very useful because it takes into account regional variability in salaries. Ask around to see if anyone might have access to this data that they are willing to share with you. Hint: post the request for this information on social media. Physician contract lawyers will also have access to this type of information – more on lawyers later.

Doximity has published physician salary information since 2017, using data from 65,000 US doctors representing 40 specialties. MedScape has been publishing data since 2011 using their database of 20,000 US doctors representing 29 specialties. These numbers are available for free and rely on self-reported information on salary, hours, location, and other work and personal details such as job challenges, benefits, gender, ethnicity, and geographic location. Some organizations, such as the veterans affairs (VA) and the federal government (search "medical officer"), provide their own free salary databases.

Ask how much other people are making, especially if you are a minority or a woman because multiple studies show that you make much less than White male peers. Even after controlling for every factor in a cohort of early career academic physicians, a 10% discrepancy between women and men remained [1]. One study found that women were already starting $16,819 behind their male colleagues with their first contract right out of residency [2]. Additionally, the Medscape Physician Compensation Report has consistently shown a racial disparity in earnings [3, 4]. While talking about money may be uncomfortable, consider that it would be better to have these conversations now than be stuck with an uncomfortable and unfair salary.

Research salaries from the resources above to have some reference points. Keep in mind that most physician contracts may have a clause saying that it is a breach of contract to disclose contents and terms of the contract. While it is probably not enforceable, protect the people sharing information with you by keeping your sources confidential. Share the numbers, because it would benefit all of us if we did this more, but keep mum about where you got them from.

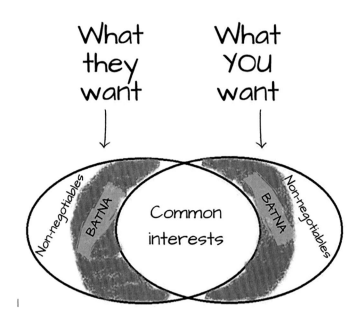

Their BATNA and Your BATNA

After you have done your research and come up with a rough idea of what work conditions and environment you want and what compensation figures you want, let's practice an important negotiation strategy. If you can't get what you want, what is your alternative?

BATNA stands for **b**est **a**lternative to a **n**egotiated **a**greement. It is a negotiation technique to get the best deal possible if your asks are not accepted. Here are possible alternative outcomes to accepting the initial job offer:

- Continue to negotiate such as for a bigger sign-on bonus. Also consider negotiating for other things that may not cost the employer much, such as a job title, but that will benefit your career goals.
- Take another job offer.
- Walk away and explore other job opportunities.

Understanding your BATNA will help you decide how aggressively you can negotiate for your asks. If you have another job offer that is equally attractive, then there is very little risk to ask for this offer to be sweeter. Even if the second job offer is not as attractive to you personally as this one (e.g., not in your ideal location), you can still leverage its benefits in negotiations. Consider also that walking away with no job might be better than accepting a job offer with many red flags and a potentially toxic environment or being stuck living in a location that you don't like. Advocate for your worth and joy.

What if the employer doesn't hire you? Can they easily hire someone else, or will they be catastrophically understaffed? What is their BATNA? Understanding the employer's alternative options will also help you better promote yourself to the employer. How will you fill their needs? How will your skills benefit them? Before the interview, network within your circle and your circle's circles to glean some details about the employer's situation and culture. During the interview, connect with staff to see if you can find out about the work culture and urgency to fill the position. Be kind, caring, and curious, and you will probably find out information that will bolster your negotiation strategy.

References

1. Jagsi R, Griffith KA, Stewart A, Sambuco D, DeCastro R, Ubel PA. Gender differences in salary in a recent cohort of early-career physician-researchers. Acad Med J Assoc Am Med Colleg. 2013;88(11):1689–99. https://doi.org/10.1097/ACM.0b013e3182a71519.

2. Lo Sasso AT, Richards MR, Chou C-F, Gerber SE. The $16,819 pay gap for newly trained physicians: the unexplained trend of men earning more than women. Health Aff. 2011;30(2):193–201. https://doi.org/10.1377/hlthaff.2010.0597.
3. Medscape Physician Compensation Report 2018. Medscape. https://www.medscape.com/slideshow/2018-compensation-overview-6009667. Date accessed: June 2, 2020
4. Medscape Physician Compensation Report 2019. Medscape. https://www.medscape.com/slideshow/2019-compensation-overview-6011286. Date accessed: June 2, 2020

Contract Considerations: Understanding the Contract

15

Joannie Yeh

Letter of Intent

After a few rounds of successful interviews, the employer may reach out to offer you the job and give you a letter of intent. Signing a letter of intent is not usually legally binding, but the specifics may vary by state and situation. Still, it is considered a sign of commitment, so do take it seriously. Before signing, negotiate as many details as possible of all your asks (which have been prepared from reading the prior chapter), and consider seeking legal advice. It's a lot cheaper and less of a hassle to change a letter of intent than it is to change a contract, so be transparent about what you want at this stage. Communicate by email or follow up with an email summary after a verbal discussion to make sure there is a paper trail in case you need to refer back to a specific detail later. Once you are satisfied with the adjustments, it's time to transfer that into a lengthy physician contract.

J. Yeh (✉)
Sidney Kimmel Medical College, Philadelphia, PA, USA

© The Author(s), under exclusive license to Springer Nature Switzerland AG 2021
P. M. Garrett, K. Yoon-Flannery (eds.), *A Pediatrician's Path*,
https://doi.org/10.1007/978-3-030-75370-2_15

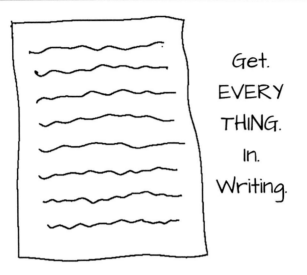

Anatomy of a Physician Contract

The physician contract often starts with a start date. Yes, even the start date should be put into writing. Get everything in writing. Don't rush yourself into starting the job if you don't have to. Consider taking some time off after residency and in between jobs to refresh. Make sure the start date fits your timeline. Also, be realistic as far as estimating how much time you will need to apply and receive relevant state licenses and to complete the credentialing process. After submitting the paperwork, expect the system to take about 3 months to process it.

The contract will specify payment information such as a base salary, qualifications for a bonus, and amount of the sign-on bonus. The bonus is often based on productivity as defined by RVUs and sometimes tied to patient satisfaction scores. Sometimes in the first contract with an employer, there is just a base salary and no bonus because it will take time to build up a patient base and generate a profit. After a few years, a new contract will include a base salary that might be less, the same, or more than the initial salary, with an opportunity to earn a bonus on an annual or quarterly basis. The sign-on bonus amount is a one-time-welcome-aboard payment and is usually tied to completion of a 2–3 year contract commitment.

The next section will usually describe your job responsibilities, call frequency, and the expected number of clinical hours per week or number of shifts per month. It will also specify which practice location you will primarily work at, especially if the employer has different offices. The contract will probably not automatically and generously include protected time for administrative duties, research, or teaching activities, so keep an eye out for that information and ask for it if you want it.

Some benefits that may be included in the contract are vacation days, parental leave, sick leave, continuing medical education days, and continuing medical education funds. The contract may also mention who is responsible for paying license fees and association memberships. Health insurance, disability insurance, and retirement benefits may not be included in contracts because the vendors that the employers use change frequently. Even if these benefits are not part of the contract, consider asking for a copy of them in writing to review.

Loan repayment may be part of the contract as well. While this seems like a wonderful perk with rising medical school debt, don't jump for joy just yet. The repayment amount may be considered taxable income and might interfere with other loan programs you might be participating with. The laws can be complicated, so it's best to consult with a contract expert and mentors who have navigated these rules themselves before agreeing to this.

The contract might specify who owns what items, entities, and information. For example, if the doctors in the practice have potential to become partners or owners, what are the requirements you have to fulfill in order to join? When equipment is purchased for the practice, who does the equipment belong to and who pays for the equipment? Will you have rights to the inventions and intellectual property that you create? Who owns the patient lists and the patient charts? While you may be at the start of your career with this contract, make sure it will also protect you when you are a few years into your career.

A major section of the contract to review very carefully is malpractice insurance, which is typically paid for by the employer. The type of malpractice insurance may be claims made or occurrence based. A claims made policy covers you for a lawsuit if it is filed and if the incident occurred while you work for the employer. A tail insurance is also needed to protect you if a lawsuit is filed after you leave the employer for an incident that occurred while you worked for the employer. The contract should note who pays for the tail insurance, you or your employer. An occurrence-based policy is usually more expensive and less commonly offered. It covers you if an incident occurred while you have the policy, even if the lawsuit is filed when you no longer have the policy and are no longer with the employer.

The length of the contract commitment is usually 2 to 3 years. The terms of termination define situations when the employer or the employee can decide to withdraw from the contract. It will also outline how much time should be given prior to withdrawing and the consequences of withdrawing. Usually, a 90-day notice is required. If you were to leave prematurely, the contract may state that you would have to pay back the sign-on bonus and to pay your own tail malpractice insurance. While no one starts their job dreaming of the day they walk away, it's important to consider and prepare for such a scenario and to make sure the terms are reasonable and not unfairly burdensome to you.

Restrictive Covenant

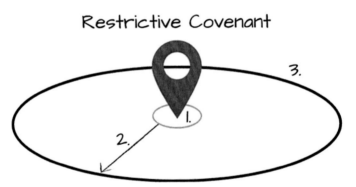

1. Practice location
2. Restrictive covenant clause restricts you from practicing within a certain radius from the practice location or locations for a certain number of years
3. Where you are allowed to practice after leaving the employer until expiration date of the clause

The restrictive covenant in the contract limits where you can work for a certain number of years after leaving the employer. This clause will specify if that distance is measured from any office owned by the employer or from the location you mostly worked at. It may also specify that it is relevant only for certain types of work. The purpose is to prevent you from taking patients away from the employer, so that means doing a similar job (e.g., hospitalist) at the hospital a few miles away is not permitted, but doing a different job (e.g., program director) might be allowed.

This is not an exhaustive description of contract terms, but the main components. Also, don't just read the contract through the lens of a happy employee. For example, what are you responsible for paying or paying back if you decide to leave before the contract duration is complete? Will you still be responsible for tail insurance if the employer terminates you without cause? Where will you be allowed to practice if you don't continue with this employer at the end contract and still want to stay local? It recommended that you talk to a local physician contract lawyer to review your first contract line by line and that you walk through various scenarios to make sure the contract is sufficient to protect your interests.

Paying for Help

This section is placed intentionally after you have been equipped to do all the work on your own. It's like how it's important to understand your taxes and review all the numbers even if you hire an accountant to file the paperwork for you. First, develop familiarity with what you want for a fulfilling career. Then, become familiar, with negotiation strategies and with how a physician contract is organized. This will save you time when you start talking to a lawyer or a negotiation service or coach. Saving time also means saving money since some services may charge an hourly rate.

Not sure if you want to invest in help? Consider that an expert-guided bump in even a few thousand dollars in salary or sign-on bonus could compound into many times that amount over years. Spending a fraction on that now for someone to help you negotiate your contract is highly recommended.

An experienced local physician contract lawyer will likely have intimate knowledge of local physician salaries and employer negotiation strategies and pain points. The lawyer can negotiate for you, as well as offer insight on what to ask for and how to counteroffer. The cost of hiring a lawyer can range from about $800 to $4000.

Physician contract negotiation and coaching services are also available to assist you with this process. The average cost is about $400. These services guide you through the offer and contract terms and assist with crafting your contract requests using regional- and specialty-specific data. They often will work with a lawyer to do a final review of the contract and answer sticky legal questions.

Review

Just to review, here is an example of the sequence of events that you might experience when looking for a job. You decide on a location and practice type. You find compatible job openings. You look up data and ask around to research the typical salary and benefits for these jobs. You interview for a couple different positions at different places and you ask curious questions. You are kind to everyone. You receive a job offer. You hire a lawyer. You counteroffer and go through a few back-and-forths until you feel that your asks have been satisfied. The employer's lawyer drafts a contract. Your lawyer and their lawyer go back and forth a few times to hash out a few other details. Finally, the contract is ready for you to sign. Congratulations!

Choosing a Career in Academic Medicine

16

Robert P. Olympia

May 5, 2017, was an important day in my academic career as it represents a lifetime of hard work and perseverance, supported by mentors, colleagues, family, and friends. The road toward promotion to Professor in the Departments of Emergency Medicine and Pediatrics at the Penn State University College of Medicine began the day I decided to become an academic pediatrician.

R. P. Olympia (✉)
Department of Emergency Medicine & Pediatrics, Penn State Hershey
Medical Center, Hershey, PA, USA
e-mail: rolympia@hmc.psu.edu

© The Author(s), under exclusive license to Springer Nature
Switzerland AG 2021
P. M. Garrett, K. Yoon-Flannery (eds.), *A Pediatrician's Path*,
https://doi.org/10.1007/978-3-030-75370-2_16

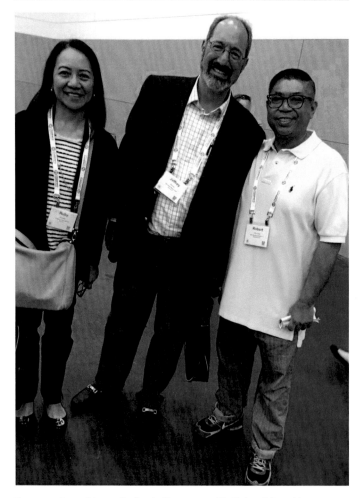

Reconnecting with my Pediatric Emergency Medicine fellowship mentors, Drs. Jeffrey Avner and Ruby Rivera, at the Pediatric Academic Societies meeting, 2019.

Pop Quiz

1. Do you consider yourself a teacher and enjoy educating and mentoring your learners?
2. Do you find satisfaction from conducting research, presenting your data at scientific meetings, or publishing your data in peer-reviewed journals?
3. Are you a lifelong learner, constantly challenging yourself to be the best clinician you can be?
4. Do you enjoy being in a leadership position or working within a team construct to serve your community or profession and improve the lives of your pediatric patients?

If you answered yes to any of these questions, you may have a future in academic pediatrics.

What Is Academic Medicine?

A career in academic medicine involves *demonstrating scholarship*, *gaining knowledge*, *and providing education*. *Demonstrating scholarship* involves imparting knowledge that results from study and research in a particular field and the dissemination of this knowledge, thus becoming an expert in a particular field. *Knowledge* is the sum or range of what is perceived, discovered, and learned over time, therefore practicing "lifelong learning." *Providing education* is the act of imparting knowledge and skill to another person/group or to cause to learn by example or experience, thus becoming a teacher and mentor.

Climbing the Academic Medicine Ladder

The goal of any academic physician is climbing the academic ladder, from Clinical Instructor to Assistant Professor to Associate Professor and ultimately Professor. Although the road may be long and difficult, at times sacrificing other nonacademic interests, in the end, the benefits and impact are numerous. While there may be nuances in the promotion and tenure process among academic institutions, criteria for promotion often involves achieving professional excellence in a combination of the following four mission areas, in accordance with your effort allocation:

- *Teaching and learning*
- *Research and creative accomplishments*
- *Patient care activities (clinical responsibilities)*
- *Service and the scholarship of service to the university, society, and the profession*

Promotion is commonly based on performance rather than time-in-rank. Performance is evaluated using the *dossier*, a standardized format for reporting activities and scholarship. Dossier reviews are conducted independently by faculty committees and administrators of each institution. Performance expectations increase as you advance in academic rank, develop mastery and independence in your field, increase scholarly accomplishments, grow your regional and national reputation, and demonstrate professional leadership. At each rung of the academic ladder, performance since the last promotion review is evaluated.

What Are the Components of a Promotion Application?

Promotion applications often include the following:

- Narrative statement (personal statement)
- External (outside your institution) evaluations
- Patient/clinical care evaluations (internal, within your institution)
- Pieces of scholarship
- Curriculum vitae
- Dossier

The *narrative statement* is usually a one- to three-page *first-person* statement about your scholarship in the context of your overall goals and philosophy, highlighting professional excellence in the four mission areas.

External evaluations are letters of recommendations from experts in your academic field/specialty, often at an academic rank higher than your current rank, from a variety of external institutions, and without a conflict of interest (i.e., no former students, teachers, mentors, colleagues, or *significant* research collaborators).

Patient/clinical care evaluations are letters of recommendation from colleagues, referring physicians, or subspecialty physicians who can comment on your clinical performance.

Pieces of scholarship are published research articles that support your overall research goals and that are cited/referenced frequently in the medical literature. Based on your academic institution, the minimum number of publications for promotion will vary, but often exclude case reports, review articles, and book chapters, and frequently require you to be the principal investigator or first author.

The format of your *curriculum vitae* (CV) will depend on your academic institution. The CV is a comprehensive record of your academic career, highlighting in a chronological fashion your involvement with the four mission areas.

The *dossier* is a record of your accomplishments in the four mission areas and is used by internal reviewers to evaluate your performance and scholarship. The information required is more detailed than a CV and must be submitted in a specific format, frequently involving colored "rainbow" folders. Four of the folders are based on the four mission areas and often include the following documentation:

1. *Teaching and learning:* (a) Lectures, seminars, courses given (both internal and external, documenting attendance numbers), (b) research supervised, (c) mentoring opportunities (students, residents, fellows, other faculty), (d) teaching evaluations (quantitative information and summary of comments), (e) peer

review of teaching (letters of recommendation from senior faculty members within your department commenting on your teaching style)

2. *Research and creative accomplishments:* (a) publications [peer-reviewed journal articles (note authorship role on each) and non-peer-reviewed publications (book editor, book chapters, review articles) including "accepted" and "in press"], (b) research projects [completed, current, planned (note role on each project), internal and external grants], (c) other creative products (e.g., educational methods or computer software developed; inventions; clinical guidelines disseminated)

3. *Patient care activities:* (a) statement of clinical assignment including time commitment and effort allocation; (b) detail on quantity and complexity of cases [patients per hour, RVU (relative value unit) productivity]; (c) quality of care (patient satisfaction data, QI activities); (d) letters from peers, colleagues, and referring physicians commenting on patient care ability and effectiveness (patient/clinical care evaluators)

4. *Service and the scholarship of service to the university, society, and the profession:* demonstrating service through committee work and leadership, both internal to your institution (in your department, in the College of Medicine, or in your hospital/health system/university) or external to your institution [within your profession (journal editorships and reviews, study sections, organizing conferences for professional associations, offices held in professional associations, government advisory groups, etc.) or within your community (citizen/client groups, outreach activities, volunteerism, etc.)].

Pearls from an Academic Climber

My journey to professor began the day I decided to become an academic pediatrician. Here are some pearls to make your journey successful:

Find your passion, seek out your niche: Do you remember why you chose pediatrics or pursued a career in your subspecialty? Allow this passion to motivate your career in academia. For me, my passion is emergency and disaster preparedness, trauma and sports medicine, access to care, and the impact of media on children. Most of my research accomplishments, education and mentorship, and patient care activities have involved these passions. I still love what I do because of these decisions.

Surround yourself with greatness: Find advisors and mentors that will guide you not only through your career in academia but also with life. I was blessed to have Drs. Magdy Attia and Jeffrey Avner train me as a resident and fellow and, even after so many years, also serve as role models and mentors throughout my career. Having an all-star team around you is better than being the only all-star.

Become a hoarder: Save letters and emails that document excellent patient care. File away lecture evaluations, and if there aren't formal evaluations for educational opportunities, develop one and collect the data. Seek letters of recommendation from learners, colleagues, or mentees who can comment on your teaching skills, mentorship abilities, or clinical acumen. It's not really hoarding if you keep things organized.

Stalk strategically: Since you will need external evaluations from "non-biased" physicians in your specialty, try to meet as many experts in your field. Go to General Pediatric and Pediatric subspecialty conferences (such as the American Academy of Pediatrics' National Conference & Exhibition or Pediatric Academic Societies annual meeting), both regionally and nationally. Introduce yourself to experts in your field, ask questions, invite them to your institution, and hand out business cards. Build your professional network; make a friend.

Keep lecturing and writing, become a scholar: Seek out educational opportunities – lectures at your institution will turn into grand rounds regionally and then expert panels nationally. Turn lectures into review articles or book chapters, turn clinical questions into research ideas, and turn quality improvement ideas into scholarship. Lectureships and publications will increase your reputation and in turn lead to multicenter research collaborations, opportunities to serve within your specialty, and means to improve the care of children globally. A laptop, pen/paper, and thinking outside the box will be your best friends.

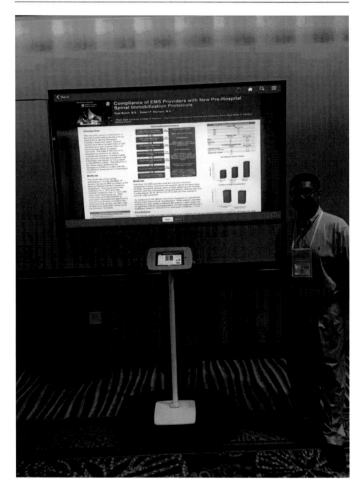

Presenting my research at the Society for Academic Emergency Medicine scientific assembly, 2017.

Delegate your work: The amount of time and effort to become promoted can be overwhelming. Utilize medical students, residents, fellows, and other colleagues in the development and implementation of research projects. Collaborate with other departments and institutions for educational and research opportunities. Make friends with the Institutional Review Board, biostatisticians, librarians, and institutional leadership and committee members. Teamwork makes the dream work.

Volunteer your time and efforts: Provide service to your department, institution, profession, and community but make sure it aligns with your passions. Do you like quality improvement? Medical education? Global health? School-based health? Whatever it may be, just get involved. And seek leadership positions if possible.

Update your CV and dossier regularly: I update my CV and dossier monthly. This may seem pathologic, but it allows me to visually see where my deficiencies lie in the four mission areas and organizes all the data that I have been hoarding over the years.

I believe my career in academic pediatrics has enriched my life, given me purpose and provided professional satisfaction, shaped the future of medicine in the learners that I have educated and mentored, and ultimately impacted the health and well-being of infants, children, and adolescents regionally, nationally, and globally. What an honor and blessing.

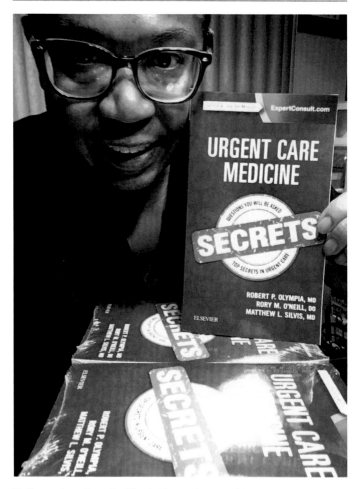

Delivery of my first edited book, Urgent Care Medicine Secrets, 2017.

Choosing a Career as a Pediatric Hospitalist

17

Ana Mann

Background

In the mid-1990s, Drs. Robert Wachter and Lee Goldman created the term "hospitalist" to refer to a new group of physicians who spent more than a quarter of their time caring for inpatients or whose primary focus was general inpatient care[1]. A hospitalist is a physician who assumes the responsibility for managing care of hospitalized patients. The hospitalists of today emerged in response to the need to replace primary care physicians, who treated their patients in all care settings, with physicians who could focus solely on the care of patients while they were in the hospital.

As is often the case, the initial reason for hiring hospitalists was financial. Medicare changed the hospital reimbursement system to a "fixed-payment" system that was based on each patient's discharge diagnosis. However, physicians continued to bill per day or per visit. In order to keep costs down, hospitals began attempting to reduce patient length of stays but were met with resistance by physicians who were used to the old system, many

---

[1] Watcher RM, Goldman L. The hospitalist movement 5 years later. *JAMA*. 2002;287(4):487-494.

A. Mann (✉)
Advocare Pediatric Urgent Care, Cherry Hill, NJ, USA

© The Author(s), under exclusive license to Springer Nature Switzerland AG 2021
P. M. Garrett, K. Yoon-Flannery (eds.), *A Pediatrician's Path*, https://doi.org/10.1007/978-3-030-75370-2_17

115

times implementing traditional 2-week inpatient recovery times independent of diagnosis. As a result, hospitals began to look for physicians whose incentives, motives, and clinical decision-making were in line with new hospital policies. They found what they were looking for in the hospitalist.[2]

Several years later, pediatrics followed suit. The emergence of pediatric hospital-based practice is relatively young. The Society of Hospital Medicine was first established in 1997 and the American Academy of Pediatrics (AAP) only recognized hospital medicine as a division with provisional status in 1999. The Academic Pediatric Association founded hospitalist medicine in 2001 and the American Board of Pediatrics (ABP) began the evaluation of potential pediatric hospitalist medicine certification status in 2016. Pediatric hospital medicine (PHM) is in an accelerated growth phase and represents one of the fastest-growing fields in US medicine with approximately 55,000 clinicians nationally.[3] Pediatric hospitalists now account for about 10% of the total hospital medicine physician workforce. Pediatric hospitalists increasingly provide important and continuous care both within free-standing children's hospitals and community-based general systems.

With the goal of raising the level of care hospitalized children receive and better defining the field, PHM successfully became a formal subspecialty. The American Board of Medical Specialties (ABMS) officially granted recognition of the American Board of Pediatrics-sponsored application for subspecialty in October of 2015.[4] Many general pediatricians still work as hospitalists, particularly in the community hospital setting. However, many are choosing to complete the 2-year fellowship and become board-certified pediatric hospitalists.

---

[2] https://journalofethics.ama-assn.org/article/hospital-medicine-movement/2008-12

[3] Wachter RM, Goldman L. Zero to 50,000: The 20th Anniversary of the Hospitalist. N Engl J Med 2016; 375:1009-1011

[4] https://www.aappublications.org/news/2016/12/14/Hospitalists121416

What Do Pediatric Hospitalists Do?

Pediatric hospitalists work in a hospital setting to take care of children, but often wear many hats. They may work in the general pediatric ward, labor and delivery, the newborn nursery, the emergency department, the neonatal intensive care unit, and the pediatric intensive care unit. Each hospitalist position brings with it different job responsibilities. Common conditions hospitalists treat include:

- Infectious illnesses of the blood, skin, lungs, and kidneys
- Respiratory illnesses such as pneumonia and croup
- Problems with chronic illnesses such as diabetes and asthma
- Common pediatric illnesses such as influenza and dehydration
- Recovery from injuries or surgeries

The patients they care for often depends on the capabilities of the hospital in which they work. For example, a hospitalist at a small community hospital would, in most instances, be able to care for a child with cellulitis, or asthma, or a urinary tract infection. But a patient with appendicitis, or in DKA, or with severe asthma might need to be transferred to a hospital with subspecialists and a PICU to care for them as needed. Many large academic hospitals have subspecialty wards that often employ hospitalists. Some hospitals may even employ a team of hospitalists that perform procedures such as conscious sedation or line placement.

In addition to the general pediatric floor, many hospitalists will also spend time doing consultations in the emergency department, evaluating newborns in the nursery, or taking care of PICU patients overnight when intensivists go home. For some, hospitalist medicine may be a natural segue from residency. They continue to take care of acutely ill/hospitalized patients, coordinate care, and perform procedures. Some pediatricians may like how the "shift" schedules of hospitalists resemble their residencies.

Hospitalist schedules vary almost as much as their job descriptions. Some doctors may work for 7 days and then have 7 days off. Some may serve as nocturnists, working only overnights. And some may have a mix of these models working a certain number of shifts per month that include both days and nights. Many physicians looking for a work-life balance may find a hospitalist position with a schedule that works for them.

As a hospitalist, you are working as part of a team that often includes nurses, pharmacists, social workers, child life specialists, nutritionists, respiratory therapists, and consulting subspecialists. There is a multidisciplinary approach to patient care and keeping open lines of communication with the entire team is an important part of the job.

Pediatric hospitalists also work closely with community pediatricians. They will keep them updated if there is a change in the child's condition and provide a summary of care and follow-up recommendations upon discharge from the hospital. The hospitalist will also coordinate subspecialty care at discharge, as needed.

Generally speaking, pediatric hospitalists are compensated at a higher rate than outpatient pediatricians.[5]

Is Pediatric Hospitalist Medicine Right for You?

Hospitalist medicine is a fast-paced and ever-evolving field. The benefits of this career include the ability to continue to do procedures, having an alternative work schedule, treating acutely ill children, and having relatively short well-defined patient encounters. For these reasons, this was the perfect job for me coming out of residency. It let me keep my skills up to date and allowed me the schedule flexibility I was seeking while caring for my young children at home. I was able to have a fulfilling career but could also be there for school functions or to volunteer in my children's classrooms.

I have always enjoyed treating sick children and I liked that my patient encounters were defined; they had a beginning, middle, and end. If you look forward to the continuity of care general pediatrics provide, this may not be the best career path for you.

---

[5] https://www.todayshospitalist.com/look-pay-shifts-pediatric-hospitalists/

Many hospitalist jobs also require at least some overnight time, so if you are not "a night person," hospitalist medicine may not be a good match. Ultimately, the overnight and weekend hours became too demanding for me and, over time, made the job less attractive. After many years I desired a more regular schedule and the luxury of sleeping in my own bed each night and eventually transitioned out of this field.

Choosing a Career in Private Practice

18

Sarah Kramer

There are many different career paths you can choose from in pediatrics. General pediatrics or fellowship? Hospitalist or private practice? Each of these could be their own chapter, so this one is about private practice in general pediatrics.

There are multiple kinds of practices. It is still possible to be a solo practitioner, but with the issues that surround insurance and billing, most private practitioners are in a group. Group practices provide several advantages over solo practice. Most importantly, you are not always on call. I remember a solo practitioner that saw newborns in the hospital where I was a resident. He finally brought on a partner and went on his first vacation in 10 years. If you are in solo practice, your phone will be attached to your hip. There are, however, ways to "join forces" with other solo practitioners to help cover each other. But in a group practice, that is built in.

In a group practice, you also always have someone to bounce things off of. No matter how long you've been in practice, something will come up that you're not sure about. It's very helpful to have other pediatricians there to ask. In my current practice, we have a great mix of seasoned and straight-out-of-residency practitioners. The new doctors tend to know the most up-to-date recommendations and protocols. Those of us who have been

S. Kramer (✉)
Watchung Pediatrics, Warren, NJ, USA
e-mail: skramer@watchungpediatrics.com

P. M. Garrett, K. Yoon-Flannery (eds.), *A Pediatrician's Path*,
https://doi.org/10.1007/978-3-030-75370-2_18

121

around longer are more used to what is seen on a day-to-day basis in outpatient pediatrics.

There are several kinds of group practices. Some are branches of a hospital practice. Others are independent of any hospital or other affiliation, like mine. And some are part of a conglomerate of practices, usually with subspecialties as well. All of them have their pros and cons, and what you choose may partially depend on what you want from a practice. If you want to be on a partnership track, then an independent group is usually the way to go. If you are not interested in being a partner, and you'd rather leave all of that to someone else, then a hospital-based or large group-based practice may be better. Generally, those pediatricians are more salaried, and while they don't have input into group decisions, they also don't have the stress of making those decisions. Part of deciding if you want to be on a partnership track involves your comfort with financial risk. There is the potential, if the practice is doing really well, to have a much bigger profit compared to the salary you would earn as an employee. However, if there are big expenses (switching to EMR, renovating an office) or if there is a down year (like right now, with COVID), then you would likely earn far less.

In my group, we have two partners/owners of the practice. The rest of us, for varying reasons, have chosen not to buy into partnership. We still attend provider meetings and give input, but ultimately it is up to the partners to make the final decision on any issues. We have expanded over the time that I have been there and currently are up to 3 offices and 17 providers. I use the term "providers" because we have both pediatricians and nurse practitioners. In my practice, the NPs function the same way we do as pediatricians. I am just as likely to ask them for help as they are to ask me! Other practices are physicians only, while others also have PAs.

In a private practice, you may have privileges at a local hospital. There are varying kinds of privileges you can have. We round on our newborns at two hospitals; we do not go to deliveries. We did admit inpatients until a few years ago, when the hospital went to a (in my opinion) very confusing computer system. Given that none of us would be in the hospital on a regular basis, we decided to turn over inpatient care to the hospitalists. (On a side note, I think that is much better, more consistent care!) So the privileges could be any combination of the above. Or your practice may not have any privileges and just have the hospitalists see the newborns as well.

When I have students with me, they always ask what a typical day looks like in the office. My day is comprised of seeing both sick and well patients. Two of our offices have primarily scheduled appointments, while the third also has sick walk-in. So it depends where I am on any given day. Usually though, I'm at one of the offices that has scheduled appointments. It can be hard to go from residency clinic, where you might see four or five patients in an afternoon, to private practice where you could see upwards of 20 in a day. We typically have a well visit scheduled every half an hour, with a sick visit on top of that. Ideally, you go in with the sick patient first, while the nurses work up the well visit. You definitely learn over time how to become more efficient and streamlined. I have the morning with patients, and then a break for lunch; but I usually make phone calls or finish the morning's charting then, if I haven't already. Sometimes we have provider meetings or lectures. The afternoon goes the same as the morning, and then I will stay after to complete any calls that need to be made that day.

Sometimes you will have to round in the hospital; most people do that in the morning, and then their day in the office starts later than usual. Walk-in is self-explanatory; you can either be beyond busy or have an hour to catch up on work.

In a private practice, you'll also almost definitely be working some weekends, and perhaps also nights. Some practices have hours on both Saturday and Sunday, some have Saturday only, and others are for emergencies only. I do think that it's rare for a practice to not have any weekend hours. You will also share holiday call with your colleagues. The nice thing about a larger practice is that you don't have to do as many weekends and holidays. I interviewed at one practice where I would have been the fourth doctor, which would result in a lot more call than I was willing to do. But you might prefer a smaller practice, which has the benefit of knowing more of the patients.

Another consideration when looking for a practice is what you are required to do on those weekends and holidays, as well as for the weekday call. Many practices have answering services with nurses who answer questions overnight. You definitely want that – or it's a lot of sleepless nights, and you've already had enough of those in residency! My current practice has set office hours on Saturday morning, with a provider rounding before going into the office and then taking calls for the rest of the day, and a provider rounding and taking calls all day on Sunday. On Sundays, we can set our own schedules, but we are expected to come in to see sick patients if necessary. The nursing service takes the calls from 6 pm to 6 am, which really helps give us some kind of a weekend, even if we're working. At a practice I used to work for, the service didn't pick up until 9 pm…then eventually 11 pm…then sometimes not at all. Having a good service is essential! You may still get calls from the hospital or nursery, but generally you can go out to dinner and get a good night's sleep.

You can also work full time or part time. In most general practices, full time is 4 days a week, plus weekends and call. In my practice, we have people working anywhere from 2 ½ to 4 full days a week, and everything in between. It's a great option to have, and you can also adjust this schedule over time, according to your needs. I was working 4 days a week until my first child was about a year old, and then I realized I needed more time for home life, so I went to 3 ½ days. That might not seem like a big drop, but it made all the difference in the world. In the current COVID environment, I've dropped back to 3 days because we don't have any childcare.

The hours you're expected to work will differ among practices as well, independent of the type of practice. Many providers are expected to work at least one late day. Some offices open earlier than others. Part of why I left my first practice was that we had to work 12-hour days twice a week, from 9 am to 9 pm. Besides being exhausted, I knew that those hours were not compatible with having a family one day, at least not for me. I took a salary cut to come to my current practice, but it was well worth it for me to not have those late hours. Practices have these hours to accommodate kids' activities and working parents' schedules, but you have to balance that with your life and your schedule. As a working parent, I'm lucky to not have to work those late hours.

The providers aren't the only part of a practice. You also need nurses and/or medical assistants to help with working up patients, doing forms, giving vaccines, and everything else that's part of the patient visit. There is also the front desk staff, office manager, and billing. Depending on your type of practice, you may or may not get to know everyone behind the scenes. Sometimes you also have ancillary providers. My practice has a phlebotomist in each office, as well as a social worker and a nutritionist who rotate between the offices. It's great to be able to provide those resources to your patients.

One important thing to remember with any practice is that it is a business and will be profit-driven. This is the case no matter what kind of practice you join. In an independent practice, the business people may be the partners you work with, but they're depending on your business to make a profit. With both independent practices and hospital-affiliated practices, there are often productivity bonuses. In my practice, it used to be more arbitrary, but in the past 3 or 4 years, we have a formula to determine our bonuses. It's nice to get a reward for squeezing in those extra patients, but you also have to decide how much of that money is worth your time. (See my chapter on burnout!) So as much as an independent practice may talk about being a "family," don't lose sight that it's a business first. I've seen the partners make changes that I don't necessarily agree with, just because some parents have made complaints. That said, there have been instances where parents have been told to leave my practice because they mistreated one of the providers, and the partners have defended the providers when parents have made unreasonable complaints.

Good billing is essential for any practice. When I started at my current practice, I realized that (a) I knew nothing about billing, (b) neither did my previous practice, and (c) they should really teach billing in residency. I had to learn about codes, modifiers, how to link diagnoses, and, most importantly, how to choose the right level of care based on the number of diagnoses, number of systems you asked about, and the length of the visit. You deserve to get paid for the time you put in!

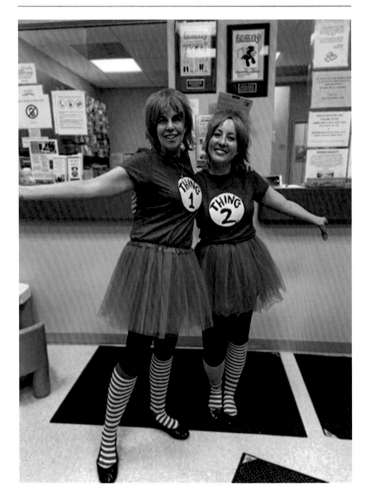

The most important thing I can tell you, though, is to go with your gut. You need to like the people you're going to work with! Do the providers seem happy? What about the nurses and front desk staff? If people are friendly and welcoming, that's a great sign. If everyone looks annoyed and miserable, well, then, it's probably not a great place to be. I think that as pediatricians, we assume that our first practice will be our "forever" practice and that one day our first patients will bring us their children to see. This is not necessarily true, and I wish I had known that when I started my career. I was at my first practice for 2 ½ years, which was probably 2 years too long. I stuck it out because I liked most of my patients, but really because it didn't occur to me that I could leave. I got to the point where I couldn't take it anymore, and there's no reason that you should put yourself through that. I've been at my current practice for more than 11 years. No place is perfect, but if you are completely miserable, know that you can find someplace else.

Choosing a Career in Public Health

19

Issy C. Esangbedo

Introduction

If you have an interest in population health or providing patient care in a safety net clinic, then working at your local public health department could be a good fit. However, there are many other opportunities within the public health sphere for pediatricians. As a clinician in a health center, you may have to tackle issues like emerging infectious diseases, racial and ethnic healthcare disparities, gun violence, child abuse, and issues around poverty like food insecurity. Delineated roles may include but are not limited to direct patient care, and you may be required to monitor the health status of patients in a community, diagnose or investigate specific health-related issues and hazards, and educate the public about health issues.

Preparing Your CV/Resume for a Public Health Job

If you can highlight any interest or experience in your CV/resume that involves working with members of the community during your pediatric residency training, that would be beneficial. Some

I. C. Esangbedo (✉)
South Philadelphia Health and Literacy Center, Philadelphia, PA, USA
e-mail: issy.esangbedo@phila.gov

© The Author(s), under exclusive license to Springer Nature Switzerland AG 2021
P. M. Garrett, K. Yoon-Flannery (eds.), *A Pediatrician's Path*,
https://doi.org/10.1007/978-3-030-75370-2_19

examples of such experiences could be lead screening in the community or BMI monitoring at a local public school. Emphasizing education or further training such as a board certification in preventive medicine, master's degree in public health, or even a degree in epidemiology could highlight your capability in data analysis and literature review. Depending on what type of job you are applying for in the public health field, you may have to customize your resume.

Work experience is always substantial, so if you have any past experience in working at a health center or similar setting in any capacity, be sure to include that in your resume. Many local health centers often provide services to new immigrants who may not be fluent in English, so proficiencies in other languages should be highlighted. Be sure to also include relevant volunteer activities that reinforce your interest in working with different underserved communities.

Job Search for a Public Health Pediatrician

There are many places to look for opportunities, but if you would like to provide primary care to an underserved population, you should start with the health department. Many major cities across the country have health departments that operate health centers. There are also federally qualified health centers (FQHCs) that are similar in operations.

1. State and local health departments:

   (i) Non-civil service physician position – Use any internet search engine (Google, Bing) to find your local health department and contact them directly.
   (ii) Civil service physician position – These positions are usually open within the health department and may not be open to the general public. Regulations vary between different local and state agencies, so you can do an internet search to see if there are any positions open to the general public at your local or state health department.

2. Federally qualified health centers: These are community-based healthcare providers that receive funds from the Health Resources and Services Administration (HRSA) Health Center Program to provide primary care services in underserved areas. You may search this website to find FQHCs in your local area and look for pediatrician openings https://findahealthcenter.hrsa.gov/.

You can also search the following websites to locate similar jobs that you may be interested in. You may have to be a member of the organization to gain access to some of these websites.

3. LinkedIn: Create a profile and highlight your experience and interests and use the job search tool – LinkedIn Jobs (https://www.linkedin.com/jobs/).
4. American Academy of Pediatrics Career Center website (https://jobs.pedjobs.org/).
5. American College of Preventive Medicine (https://www.acpm.org/?page=CareerCenter). These job postings are open to those pediatricians certified in preventive medicine.
6. American Public Health Association (https://www.apha.org/professional-development/public-health-careermart).
7. Centers for Disease Control (https://www.cdc.gov/employment/recruitment/).
8. Federal Government – General Employment (https://www.usajobs.gov).

Interviewing for the Job

Do your research. If you are interested in employment at your local health department, then it is important to be aware of their mission and the major health problems facing the community. The selection process usually favors candidates that have exhibited a desire to make a significant contribution to the well-being and safety of the members of the community as evident in their education, work, and volunteer experience, for example, pediatricians that have shown an interest in public health issues like childhood immunizations, lead poisoning in children, obesity, and food insecurity.

Getting invited for an interview means that there is a strong interest in your application, and the interview is to determine if the candidate's expectations meet that of the employer and vice versa.

Negotiating Contracts and Medical Liability Insurance

Public health careers with the state and local health departments offer competitive salaries and many benefits. Civil service physician positions are usually attained through the Civil Service Merit System, and these positions provide comprehensive health insurance benefits, retirement benefits, generous leave programs, and job security. State and local governmental employees have to take civil service examinations to get opportunities for career advancement and transfer positions.

Remuneration is usually not negotiable because all clinicians with similar job descriptions at the health department are paid at the same rate. Civil service positions may have additional benefits like participation in pension programs, but salary is the same as non-civil service positions. Negotiations for salary increases and benefits are usually handled by union representatives for the entire workforce. Medical malpractice insurance is covered by the health department, and the type of coverage depends on your health department. Many health departments will provide occurrence coverage or claims-made with an included extended reporting period (ERP) or tail coverage.

Starting Your New Position

All new employees typically have about a 6-month probationary period before being awarded permanent employment status when working for the local government, and this applies to the health department. You will have a performance report with your supervisor during this time frame to determine if you will be granted a permanent status or separated from the position.

There are many opportunities for continuing education and staff development training. State and local health departments organize regular meetings and conferences for employees to remain current on topics in public health and their individual fields. Depending on the institution tuition benefits, professional conference leave and other programs may be available to facilitate continuing medical education.

Choosing a Career in Pediatric Urgent Care

20

Ana Mann

Introduction

Every pediatrician has received that 8 pm call from a parent whose child cannot stop screaming and is tugging at their ear. For a long time, pediatricians were able to give parents two options: try some pain medicine and call the office in the morning for an appointment or go the emergency department. Pediatric urgent care facilities now provide a third option.

Pediatric urgent care facilities are becoming increasingly common across the country. They fill a void for concerned parents that need their child seen soon for things that do not require an emergency room visit.

Urgent care (UC) is one of the fastest-growing venues of healthcare delivery used to treat many nonemergent conditions [1]. Urgent care, as defined by the American College of Emergency Physicians, is a walk-in clinic focused on the delivery of medical care for minor illnesses and injuries in an ambulatory medical facility outside of a traditional hospital-based or freestanding emergency department [2]. These centers are distinct from a hospital emergency department, doctor's office, or clinic. Previous

A. Mann (✉)
Advocare Pediatric Urgent Care, Cherry Hill, NJ, USA

P. M. Garrett, K. Yoon-Flannery (eds.), *A Pediatrician's Path*,
https://doi.org/10.1007/978-3-030-75370-2_20

135

studies have cited the accessibility, ease of use, timeliness of visits, and decreased cost as reasons patients are increasingly visiting these sites [3].

The American Academy of Pediatrics (AAP) endorses UC as a "safe, effective adjunct to, but not a replacement for, the medical home or emergency department" [4]. These lower-acuity sites have been shown to provide care of comparable quality to care delivered in the emergency department (ED) setting for appropriate cases [5].

Two areas in which the urgent care clinic concept excels are convenience and cost. Pediatric urgent care clinics are convenient because they almost always offer shorter wait times than emergency rooms, and they are often directly associated with a patient's pediatric primary care provider, so they can provide "continuity of treatment" and follow-up. Additionally, you are less likely to incur massive out-of-pocket expenses, the high co-pays and "surprise charges" that often result from a late-night visit to an emergency room.

Who Should Visit a Pediatric Urgent Care Center?

Most pediatric urgent care centers are equipped to diagnose and treat a wide variety of complaints. Pediatric urgent care focuses on providing acute assessment, management, and treatment of mild-moderately sick or injured kids, with an emphasis on rapid service and providing a harmonious, nonthreatening environment at low cost. These include the following:

Infections of the ear, eye, skin, and urinary tract	Sore throat	Fever	Headaches
Mild breathing problems	Lacerations	Strains/sprains/ fractures	Foreign body removal
Asthma flares	Flu-like illness/ URI/croup	Mild burns	Vomiting/ diarrhea/ dehydration

These are only a few of the many conditions a pediatric urgent care is equipped to treat. A mild/moderate asthmatic may get the therapy they need to safely go home. A child with a chin laceration can have it repaired.

Most pediatric urgent care centers also have X-ray capabilities on site so patients can get X-rays and be splinted appropriately. Some may even offer IV fluids for patients with mild/moderate dehydration who continue to have symptoms despite oral medication. Conversely, if a child comes in and is too sick for treatment in urgent care, the physician is also prepared to stabilize the patient and transfer them to an emergency department as soon as possible.

Is a Career in Pediatric Urgent Care Right for You?

Pediatric urgent care centers are often staffed by pediatric-trained physicians and nurses. In addition, staff can often include a secretary, medical assistants, and radiology technologists. Physicians working in a pediatric urgent care facility are often using the same skills used in outpatient, hospital, and emergency department settings.

While they are commonly diagnosing and treating fevers, respiratory illnesses and asthma exacerbations, they are also performing laceration repairs, foreign body removals, incision and drainage of abscesses, and splinting of fractures. For this reason, this career is ideal for physicians that still enjoy being "hands-on" and performing procedures.

In addition to evaluating and treating patients, pediatric urgent care physicians are also communicating with patients' primary doctors to ensure proper follow-up and continuity of care.

Most pediatric urgent care centers are open during off hours and act as a supplement to traditional pediatric practices. They are often open in the early morning or late into the evening. These "off hours" may be attractive for some physicians who want to maintain a home/life balance.

Pediatric urgent care facilities are increasingly providing a valuable service to children and their families by remaining open after their pediatricians' offices have closed and providing services that previously required a visit to the emergency room.

As a physician working in the hospital setting for most of my career, transitioning to pediatric urgent care was a natural next step for me. I was able to continue treating acutely ill children and performing procedures. In addition, I was able to be home with my family most mornings, then work in the afternoons/evenings when my urgent care center opened. Unlike hospital work, there were no overnight hours, which was one of my major considerations for leaving hospital medicine. The job brings a lot of satisfaction and, for me, struck a great balance between hospital and outpatient pediatric practice.

References

1. Boyle M. The Healthcare Executive's Guide to Urgent Care Centers and Freestanding EDs. HealthLeaders Media. 2012. Available at: http://healthleadersmedia.com/supplemental/10444_browse.pdf.
2. https://www.acep.org/patient-care/policy-statements/urgent-care-centers/.
3. Weinick RM, Betancourt RM. No appointment needed: the resurgence of urgent care centers in the United States. Oakland: California HealthCare Foundation; 2007. Available at: http://www.chcf.org/~/media/MEDIALIBRARYFiles/PDF/PDFN/PDFNoAppointmentNecessaryUrgentCareCenters.pdf.
4. Conners G, Committee on Pediatric Emergency Medicine. Pediatric care recommendations for freestanding urgent care facilities. Pediatrics. 2014;133(5):950–3.
5. Mehrotra A, Liu H, Adams JL, et al. Comparing costs and quality of care at retail clinics with that of other medical settings for 3 common illnesses. Ann Intern Med. 2009;151(5):321–8.

Choosing a Career in Direct Primary Care

21

S. Amna Husain

Thinking Outside the Box: Direct Primary Care and Concierge Medicine

The term "concierge medicine" definitely has an allure to it, but what does it mean? Where do you get started? How feasible is it to practice outside the traditional insurance model? You may have also heard of the term "direct primary care" or simply DPC. Direct primary care is quickly becoming a popular option for pediatricians to optimize work-life balance, patient satisfaction, and your own professional satisfaction. Both concierge medicine and DPC can be considered niche markets that have been slowly increasing in number for the last 10 years. They offer physicians flexibility and chances of success both in rural and urban communities as they can be customizable.

Definition of Direct Primary Care (DPC)

Direct primary care (DPC) is a unique medicine model that allows patients a more personalized experience without the typical limitations of health insurance like shorter appointments, longer wait

S. A. Husain (✉)
Pure Direct Pediatrics, Marlboro, NJ, USA
e-mail: dr.amnahusain@gmail.com

© The Author(s), under exclusive license to Springer Nature Switzerland AG 2021
P. M. Garrett, K. Yoon-Flannery (eds.), *A Pediatrician's Path*,
https://doi.org/10.1007/978-3-030-75370-2_21

periods, etc. Called subscription-based healthcare by some, this model of care is arguably higher quality at a reasonable cost. At the core of DPC, patients pay a fixed monthly fee *directly* to their primary care doctor. In the case of a pediatric practice, the parents pay a fixed monthly fee to the pediatrician that will encompass their child's pediatric care for that monthly fee. As the owner and physician of the DPC practice, you can choose to include what services are included and what would fall outside the fixed monthly fee's services. DPC models bypass the third party insurance companies that currently pay for primary care. Of course, it is up to the patients if they choose to remain insured. Not only as a medical health care professional but also a parent, I highly encourage families to keep insurance. Patients can maintain insurance to cover medications, labs, imaging, and subspecialist fees but also what insurance was meant to cover: bad, expensive medical problems that might or might not happen to you or your family. The saying goes "you're healthy until you're not," and insurance can help with sky-high hospitalization and imaging bills should they arise. However, good insurance *does not* equal good healthcare.

Who Would This Model Work For?

The beauty of DPC is this works for anyone who needs a primary care physician! This model doesn't mesh with fields that collaborate and work within the hospital (OB-GYN, hospitalists, surgical or heavy procedure fields). Insurance is intricately involved in the hospital or inpatient side, so setting and paying cash pay fees for a surgery isn't feasible for the majority. What we know now is the relationship between insurance reimbursement and *outpatient* primary care doesn't run smoothly, to say the least. Revenues are lower and lower, driving physicians to see more and more volume, which disrupts patient and physician satisfaction and increases rates of physician burnout.

How does DPC help the patient? Right now, patients are frustrated. They're frustrated with short, rushed appointment times, difficulty communicating with the office, long wait periods to get an appointment see their personal physician, and long waiting room times.

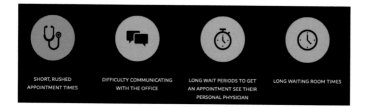

They're frustrated with Western medicine which they feel dismisses their thoughts, input, opinions, and feelings. In reality, most physicians are practicing medicine to the best of their ability; they are simply extremely strapped for time and have less autonomy over how they choose to schedule their patients.

Wasn't primary care about continuity of care and the ability to respond to patients' questions? With today's current busy outpatient schedules for physicians, this isn't feasible.

With DPC, primary care is no longer volume driven, it's "value driven." Under the monthly membership fee, you determine your value and provide care that is convenient for the patient, not just the doctor or "the system." You have the ability to include services that you like with 100% price transparency, so patients will always know the value of their care by you, the physician. Depending on where you live and the number of uninsured patients you see, you can provide negotiated cash lab and imaging pricing. Thinking outside of the box and stepping away from "the system," you begin to appreciate the finer aspects of medicine – the way medicine used to be practiced, unrushed office visits, 30–60 minutes in length with no copayments. You have the ability to offer house calls, the way doctors once used to before red tape stepped in.

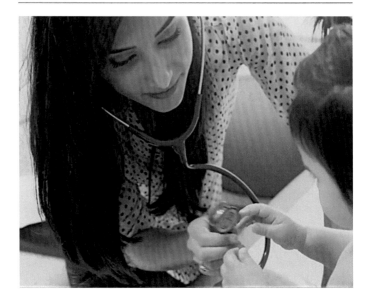

Personally, my favorite aspect is texting, phone, and email access to your doctor. As a mother, I understand most millennial parents today turn to the internet, leading to either more fear or irrelevant fake medical advice. Some parents call their office hours at ungodly times with non-emergent questions, simply thinking their insurance is "paying for it." We know that's simply not true. No, typically, when we take that 4-am call about Tylenol dosing, we are *not* being compensated.

By adding a value to your services, you'll find that patients actually only reach out to you if there's a true issue, and when they do so, most of the time, they're more respectful of your time and appreciative of your advice. They won't need to turn to the internet or their Facebook mom groups because they can text their board-certified doctors' pictures of rashes instantly. The patient communicates directly with his or her doctor, no answering service. That can be a lot to swallow for some doctors which is why we'll discuss the pros and cons of DPC medicine for physicians.

How Does DPC Help the Physician?

Let me provide you a little back story on myself. I completed residency in 2018. I always envisioned myself in the private practice realm…part-time initially, but as my children grew, I had more time to dedicate to my role as a general outpatient pediatrician. I would expand my role in the private practice and work full-time, perhaps buying in to become a partner or an associate. After I sat for my boards (and passed!), I began seriously looking for pediatric jobs, and to be blunt, I was utterly underwhelmed. The pickings were slim; the salaries even slimmer. The schedules offered didn't work with my physician husband who was starting his own practice. I had a 6-month-old at home, so having a dependable schedule for balancing child care mattered. I know I'm not the only doctor who has had these struggles. Many of you can relate to one of these issues. I had heard of DPC, but thought there was no way I could start my own practice, fresh out of residency…Could I?

Spoiler alert: I did. I single-handedly started the first pediatric DPC in my state. I broke it down for myself very simply: Would I rather see a lot of patients and spend less time with them, or see less patients and spend more time with each one? Was it quantity or quality that mattered to me? Did I really want to work for someone else? Now, many employers can be absolute joys to work with. I didn't encounter that on my job search. I encountered misogyny, bullying, and that "gut feeling" telling me not to take the job. The other item that drove me toward DPC was the flexibility: complete control over my income, my schedule, and autonomy with medical decision-making. If you're working in a practice where the patient scheduling, referral process, or work flow isn't working, are you able to speak up and express your unhappiness and propose quality initiatives to improve measures? In my own practice, I could tailor it to fit mine and my patients' needs.

Sounds amazing, right? Then why isn't *everyone* doing this? There's a reason; this is *hard*. You need to have the entrepreneurial spirit to grind and be patient until you are successful. I do *not* think this path is for everyone at least now. Maybe in 10 years with more acceptance of the concept, definitely, but right now in 2020, you need to ask yourself some tough questions.

"Do you still 'like' your job?" Are you ready to walk away from a job that still brings you some level of satisfaction? If you begin your own DPC practice, will that solve your burnout or is it time to move away from your career in medicine?

"Are you ok with a pay cut?" I won't lie. There is a financial risk involved. Typically, it takes 2–3 years with minimal to no income. In general, that's how long it takes any practice to determine viability. But DPC is trickier as the model is less well known, and patient panels can fill slowly.

"Are you able to run your own business, from A to Z and more?" I'm talking book keeping, inventory, IT, scheduling, the works.

Last but not least, remember *you are delivering an experience*. You're not reinventing the wheel here. You are bringing medicine back, the way it used to be practiced, but into the digital age. Owning your own practice comes with headaches but also perks. You can give your DPC practice whatever flavors you want. For example, in addition to being a board-certified pediatrician, I'm also a licensed and boarded lactation consultant, so my practice is very heavy in breastfeeding medicine. I also focus more on pediatric nutrition and mental health in my well checks and sick visits, which works well with the longer appointment times and close-knit medical home the pediatric DPC promotes.

This chapter started out discussing concierge care, and I purposely put off answering what it means because it's a very broad and generalized term. Both the concierge and the DPC models have membership fees paid by the patient. However, traditionally, concierge practices may also bill the patient's insurance company for covered services, while the DPC practice usually relies solely on the membership fees to cover costs. Typically, concierge service practices only do well in highly affluent urban regions, but DPC practices can function well in rural areas as well. Some DPC proponents are incredibly passionate about how DPC differs sharply from concierge medicine, stating DPC monthly fees are typically cheaper or concierge practices' monthly fees encompass a broader range of services. Others say labelling yourself as "concierge" commits you to a level of care and availability that is and will always be expected by the patient. Personally, I feel pediatric DPC can't exist without some degree of concierge medicine, by nature and needs of our patients and their parents/caregivers.

Writing this now in 2020, the year that COVID has affected so many physicians' lives and livelihoods, I'm grateful to be my own employer. Rather than patients leaving my DPC practice viewing it as a "luxury," more have joined, understanding the value of science-backed evidence and the importance of a medical physician. There have certainly been struggles as well, especially as a small business owner managing during a pandemic.

If you're a physician considering either DPC or concierge models, congratulations on stretching your mind and beginning to think outside the box and considering a different path! This path is certainly not for everyone, but if I could pass on some parting advice it would be: Once you make a decision, commit and believe in yourself. Owning your own business, practicing medicine on your own terms, along with autonomy and branding may bring even more opportunities to your door than you ever expected.

. . .

"The real test is not whether you avoid failure, because you won't. It's whether you let it harden or shame you into inaction, or whether you learn from it; whether you choose to persevere." – Barack Obama

Nonclinical Roles

22

Krupa Playforth

Introduction

As a graduating resident, it is very easy to pigeonhole yourself into believing that clinical medicine is your only option moving forward (or to assume you do not have the skills needed to succeed in another area). This is simply not the case. Physicians are in high demand across numerous careers; we have great work ethic, have been trained to learn quickly and work efficiently under pressure, and are able to think critically. These skills are valuable!

Is a Nonclinical Job the Right Pathway for You?

Deciding on a career path requires a deep understanding of your professional goals, life priorities, and skills. What makes a job or task rewarding for you? What compromises are you willing to make? It is also important to understand why you are seeking a transition. The best reason to transition to a nonclinical career is if this will help you achieve those personal or career goals, which could include improved work-life balance, compensation (especially in comparison to pediatric general practice), or obtaining additional leadership or job opportunities.

K. Playforth (✉)
The Pediatrician Mom, Mclean, VA, USA
http://www.thepediatricianmom.com/

In most cases, nonclinical jobs will offer some of these benefits. On the other hand, these jobs may require more travel, deadlines, and pressure, and some physicians describe them as monotonous in comparison to the diversity of patient care.

In discussing nonclinical job opportunities with those who have made the transition, there are two common themes: clinical experience and networking. Almost all these jobs prefer to hire physicians with clinical experience, so in most cases, I recommend working in a clinical setting for several years before applying. Your understanding of clinical medicine will make you a far more competitive candidate for a nonclinical career. Reaching out to other physicians who work in these fields will help you understand what the day-to-day of their job is like (and how it differs from clinical practice). Making these connections also helps you to stay updated regarding jobs that become available in your field of choice.

Some Examples of Nonclinical Jobs

Utilization Management/Physician Advisor Role

Physicians who work in these areas are effectively stewards of the system. The job primarily consists of reviewing charts to evaluate the patient's workup. One can work either with insurers (referred to as UM or utilization management) or with hospitals (often as a consultant with an independent firm, referred to as a physician advisor).

Physicians who work in UM conduct chart reviews to ensure a patient received cost-effective and appropriate care, in the right setting. Physician advisors review charts to ensure documentation and decision-making complies with utilization and quality regulations, sometimes helping hospitalists make decisions regarding evidence-based care, as well as the length and type of admission. They sometimes play a role in quality improvement on a hospital-wide basis. Physician advisors can serve as liaisons with insurance companies, helping conduct peer-to-peer reviews.

A physician who is excellent at analytical thinking will thrive in this type of career. Many find the option to work from home appealing, with more predictable standard business hours and a good deal more flexibility. However, this work can be quite dry and monotonous. For both UM and physician advising, preference tends to be given to physicians with experience as hospitalists. Salaries range depending on the size of the company and the role, but a ballpark for a starting salary would be in the 200,000–250,000 range. There are also bonuses, standard benefits, and opportunities for job growth and advancement.

Making connections with physicians who are already working in these roles is an important step to finding openings and learning more about the job itself. LinkedIn and recruiters can also help. For someone who is detail-oriented and passionate about appropriate resource management, these are excellent nonclinical career options.

Government/Regulatory Work

Working for governmental organizations such as the FDA or the NIH offers an array of opportunities, but options can be limited by where you live. Physicians can contribute to basic science research, regulatory work, or policy development, depending on their interests. Although you may worry that you do not have the background or skills necessary to work in this field, these organizations are large and typically have well-developed training programs to teach necessary skills over the first few years of employment.

The work is intellectually stimulating and offers leadership and growth opportunities for those who are interested. For those with family commitments, having predictable (but often flexible) hours is appealing, and like many other government jobs, they typically offer great benefits. With that said, priority is given to physicians with several years of clinical experience, and pay scales and promotions are strictly standardized. Much of this type of work is team-based, with contributions from professionals in various fields, and it often attracts physicians who are mid-to-late career.

Although it is possible to find many of these jobs advertised on usajobs.gov, openings may not be listed immediately. For that reason, networking with physicians already working in your area of interest can be helpful for learning about job opportunities (and may well help expedite some of the process, which can be quite slow).

Pharma/Biotech Industry

Jobs in the pharma and biotech fields are diverse. Physicians who have transitioned to these roles often find the option of being involved in drug development from the very beginning to be very rewarding. Those that are interested in research can help design protocols, while physicians who are very analytical and detail-oriented may be more interested in pharmacovigilance and reviewing safety data. Some physicians enjoy participating in the business or education aspects of pharma.

Strong interpersonal skills are highly valued because you will work closely with professionals from various backgrounds (sales, bench research, marketing) on the same projects. Many of these companies typically prefer to hire physicians with experience in clinical practice because of their perspective and their credibility when it comes to marketing and engaging with other physicians.

Careers in the pharma/biotech industries are generally very intellectually stimulating and rewarding with the potential for national or even global impact. The career provides many ongoing learning opportunities because you are likely to work on products across multiple specialties, which provides many ongoing learning opportunities over the course of your career. These careers are well-reimbursed (although the specifics depend on your role), but a ballpark starting salary would be $200,000–250,000 with a strong bonus structure that can range from 15 to 45% of your annual salary, along with stock options.

Depending on your role, travel may be required, and it is often more challenging to work part-time. Additionally for some physicians, the hierarchies, bureaucracy, and decision-making strategies can be an adjustment.

Consulting and Administration

Consulting can take many forms. The healthcare industry is highly profitable and constantly expanding, so consulting firms are often interested in hiring physicians who can provide a clinical perspective to help develop solutions to various problems. For example, healthcare information technology and electronic medical record software design are rapidly growing fields, and physicians who have practiced clinical medicine can provide valuable input to help develop and market new products. Physician consultants sometimes work with pharmaceutical companies, health insurance companies, investment firms, and even law firms to provide medical expertise and to interface with medical-based clients who may be more receptive to information from a clinician.

If you are interested in pursuing a consulting career, it may be worth obtaining experience in quality improvement activities in your office or hospital. Physician consultants need to be able to work effectively with professionals from various backgrounds, including other physicians, hospital staff, and administrators. They need to be great communicators, with good attention to detail. These jobs typically require travel but are well reimbursed and rewarding.

Writing and Media

Many physicians are talented writers who are looking to explore the field of medical writing, which can be quite diverse. A medical background is helpful for understanding and presenting medical concepts and terminology. Regulatory medical writers put together scientific/technical reports or other material required for the approval of drugs and other products. Educational medical writers put together teaching material, articles for journals, or promotional packets targeting a variety of audiences. Some physicians may also choose to work as freelancers.

Pharmaceutical and other research companies are often interested in hiring physicians, as are companies that put together tests and CME presentations. Of course, for those interested in more traditional journalism, many media sources have healthcare correspondents as part of their team. The advantages of this type of career lie in flexibility and the option to work from home. This may be less true as a journalist because of the need to travel.

To get started in medical writing, you need to write! Develop a portfolio of writing samples that showcase your abilities as a writer and consider submitting these to existing publications. The American Medical Writers Association (AMWA) is also a great resource with forums for networking and courses that teach the nuances of medical writing. Ultimately the financial return for these careers is very variable and depends on exactly which path you pursue. Breaking into medical writing can be challenging and takes persistence. Plan to start small, hone your writing skills, and build your brand.

How to Start Looking for a Nonclinical Career

As discussed above, networking is key to pursuing many of these nonclinical opportunities. Mentoring relationships are a valuable way to make connections, learn more about job specifics, and learn about the open positions. Many physicians join online or Facebook groups to connect with mentors, and these are actually a great resource for job listings as well.

Summary

Many physicians make the mistake of feeling trapped by their career choice. Clinical medicine is not for everyone. Your experience and knowledge base as a physician can be applied in many spheres: public health, occupational health, teaching, and medical writing. The key is to recognize that those options exist and that your medical degree and residency experience expand, rather than limit, your options. The careers discussed in this article are only a fraction of the options, and mentoring relationships are a valuable way to make connections, learn more about job specifics, and learn about job openings.

Resources

Websites

Nonclinicaldoctors.com
Lookforzebras.com
Usajobs.gov
Amwa.org
Docjobs.com

Books 50 Nonclinical Careers for Physicians: Fulfilling, Meaningful, and Lucrative Alternatives to Direct Patient Care (by Sylvie Stacy, MD, MPH).

Part III

After Finding a Job

Moving (For Your First Big-Kid Job!)

23

Jaime Jump

Introduction

You did it! Congratulations! Whatever the length of your training, it can feel like a never-ending, uphill journey. Moving happens during many phases of our medical training (medical school to residency, residency to fellowship); however, the intent of this chapter is to focus on moving after the acceptance of your first attending job.

The job search itself is incredibly challenging and geography definitely becomes a topic of interest as residency/fellowship training comes to an end. Some of your friends and colleagues will be lucky enough to find their dream job in their desired location. Sometimes, however, you have to start over in a new zip code. Moving is an overwhelming task that requires planning and foresight to be done under the least amount of stress possible. I hope to provide a little bit of framework to help address the moving process and some of the issues that may pop up during the process given my own cross-country relocation experience.

J. Jump (✉)
Baylor College of Medicine, Houston, TX, USA

Sections of Critical Care and Palliative Care, Texas Children's Hospital, Houston, TX, USA
e-mail: jxjump@texaschildrens.org

Show Me the Money

After you complete your training, you have a lot on your plate. You have probably envisioned graduating, signing your job contract, moving into a house without IKEA furniture, and finally working as an independent physician. Easy right? Unfortunately, you immediately have another to-do-list not to mention moving is a very expensive undertaking. Whether you realize it or not, you have become pretty money savvy after many years of living on a trainee salary. However, before you start budgeting and putting aside money for all of your moving expenses, you need to discuss whether or not it is possible to negotiate moving expenses into your job contract. Many academic institutions and private practices will allot 5000–10,000 dollars for all moving-related expenses, especially for geographically distant relocations. Even if you are not able to negotiate the moving expenses into your contract, it is often smart to also factor in many other items into your budget including licensure applications, board exam fees, and insurance costs. None, some, or all of these items may be reimbursed after your employment start date. Make sure to save all of your receipts and keep them in an easily accessible folder or file on your computer. You will need all of your receipts for institution reimbursement. It is also important to be prepared for some miscellaneous expenses that may include things like a mortgage down payment and utility disconnection and reconnection fees.

Many of us choose to take some time off in between ending our training and starting our new job. You will still need health insurance! Make sure to pick up COBRA or have another health insurance backup until your new benefit coverage period begins. It would also be prudent to think about how you will handle your student loan payment with a lag in income. Some of these matters tend to be an afterthought and can cause more headaches during an already stressful time.

Buy or Rent?

When choosing to relocate, it is often difficult to decide if you should immediately look into purchasing a home or you should choose to rent for a period of time while you adjust to living in a new city. As you can imagine, this decision is highly personal and depends on your family circumstances. To give you an example, I was moving cross-country with three big dogs. I knew that finding a place to rent in that situation would be much more difficult, and I chose to purchase a home.

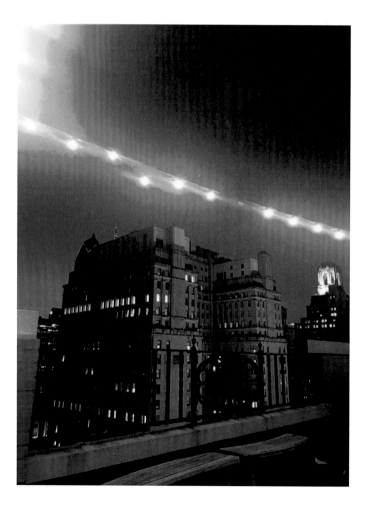

The advantage of renting when you move to a new city is that you can really explore and get to know the area before committing to a home purchase. You may be surprised that your commute is longer than expected or that the schools are much better in a different area. Over time, you will become more comfortable in your new city before you commit to a more permanent living situation. Relocating for a job can also come with the risk of not liking your new job or your new zip code. Many sources estimate that about half of new physicians will leave their first job within 1–3 years. Renting gives some extra security in this scenario as the costs for breaking a lease will likely be much less than having to turn around and sell your recently purchased home.

On the flip side, purchasing a home does have its advantages as well. Purchasing a home allows you to start over in a place that you can call your own. Some people are overwhelmed with the potential of having to move into a new home after renting. Purchasing a home allows you to only make the big move one time. If you are moving with a significant other and/or children, settling into a more permanent residence may also help them to settle into their new job, school, and routine in their new neighborhood.

Who Are You Going to Call?

If you are fortunate enough to negotiate your moving expenses into your contract, definitely go with professional movers. Some academic institutions and private practices have specific moving companies that they work with routinely and can recommend. Even if you have to bear the cost of the move yourself, you are moving a long distance, or you are moving a large household with lots of moving parts including large pieces of furniture and household items, I would also budget for a professional moving company. If you aren't able to obtain any personal or professional references for a professional moving company, do your homework and make sure to read customer reviews. Companies that lack transparency surrounding timelines and the care of your possessions can lead to a lot of frustration. Dishonest companies have been known to increase the cost to you for longer holding of your items when they fail to deliver them within the negotiated time-line.

A reputable moving company will typically schedule an appointment with you to assess the volume of items that you will need to move and will provide you with an estimate (all things included boxing, taping, etc.). Make sure to inquire about any special promotions they may have running, especially in the set-ting of a large-volume move. If you are considering shipping a vehicle, it is also important to discuss this with the same company for ease of tracking. Remember that you have consumer rights and discuss their policies surrounding loss or damage of items during the moving process.

Tackling a short move with a smaller number of items may allow for you to manage your own move. In this scenario you can set the schedule and the time. You can also organize and pack all of your belongings the way that you prefer which may potentially lead to a faster and more efficient unpacking process. The same rules apply to rental companies in terms of doing your homework and holding the company to certain standards. Do your best to try not to get price gouged for essential moving supplies like boxes and tape purchased at the rental company. Try to be creative and ask your local grocery store or retail stores if they have any left-over boxes that you can have. Use these boxes for packing when you can, it can potentially save you a few hundred dollars!

Moving Survival Essentials

You are bound to pack some essentials that may take a few weeks to arrive at their final destination. Make a list of things that you need to have with you at all times for survival. Pack a suitcase like you are preparing for a 1- to 2-week vacation. It is also important to plan out how you will survive the first weeks while you are unpacking in your new home. Plan for where you will sleep until your bed arrives, bring bathroom essentials (shower curtain, tow-els, toilet paper) and kitchen essentials (some silverware, a few cups, plates, and bowels), and keep out some tools to use for odd jobs that will come up. The goal is to make sure you can survive relatively comfortably until the moving company arrives with all of your belongings. It can take 4–6 weeks for a professional moving company to deliver all of your items. Make sure to try to time this appropriately so that you are ready and able to supervise the unloading of all of your stuff. You should also try to assess for any potential damage that occurred to your belongings during the move. Take a picture, and review the moving company policies surrounding reimbursement or replacement of damaged or broken items.

Other Chores

The relocation to-do list is long. Itemize your list of personal and professional to-dos in order of priority. Keep all of your on-boarding paperwork in an online or paper folder, and have things accessible at all times. Make sure to keep in touch with your new employer about any requirements that have not been completed, so that you can ensure you are credentialed and ready to start work by your anticipated start date. Personal to-do lists may also include things such as opening a new bank account and obtaining a new state driver's license and car registration.

Take-Home Thoughts

Moving is hard and there are a lot of moving parts. Try to keep things in perspective and focus on the end goal. Not everything has to get done in 1 day!

– Do your homework and hire a reputable moving company.
– Prioritize and organize your to-do list.
– Enlist help (any and all takers).
– Let the professionals take care of all the little details (and try to enjoy the ride, literally!).

Licenses, Credentials, and Privileges

24

Nicole Streeks-Wooden

Introduction

Hooray! You are seeing the light at the end of the pediatric residency tunnel and have sealed the deal on your first real pediatrician job or have decided to further specialize! Be sure to celebrate this momentous achievement and then prepare yourself to start obtaining all the tools you need to actually be able to get the job done.

N. Streeks-Wooden (✉)
Pediatrics, CAMCare Health Corporation, Camden, NJ, USA

© The Author(s), under exclusive license to Springer Nature Switzerland AG 2021
P. M. Garrett, K. Yoon-Flannery (eds.), *A Pediatrician's Path*,
https://doi.org/10.1007/978-3-030-75370-2_24

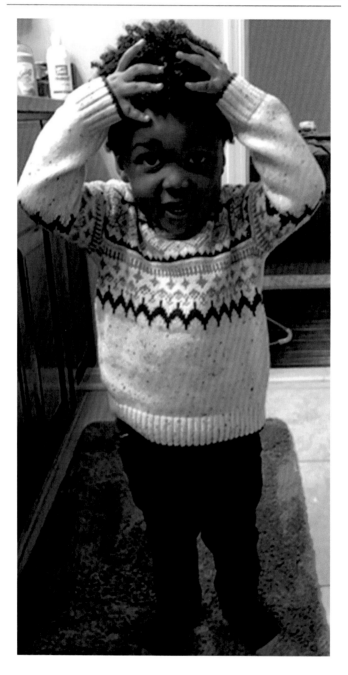

Licenses

This is the document that allows you to freely make all of those attending decisions independently and sign your notes without all of those attestations! (*Some of you may already have obtained your unrestricted medical license due to allowances in the state for which you trained.*) For those of you that are choosing to go into fellowship, obtaining an unrestricted medical license in your fellowship state may still be helpful for any future moonlighting opportunities. For the rest of you, around about 6 months before your end of residency (or whenever you land the job), start your medical license application. Go ahead and stop by your residency coordinators office (or have their contact information readily available), as they can be a great resource for document collection for many of the necessary requirements for your applications. If your employer didn't specifically mention it during the interview process, now is also a good time to discuss any current/future plans to practice in a nearby state, where you will also need a license (e.g., many people who work in the **DC-M**aryland-**V**irginia areas have satellite offices/hospital affiliations across state or city lines, or some who work in Philadelphia, Pennsylvania, may also work in Southern New Jersey). Once you know what state/states you'll be applying in, verify with your employer if there is any reimbursement for expenses paid for licensing. If there is, then you can keep all of your receipts for submission! Some employers may not specifically reimburse you for the license but will allow you to use CME (continuing medical education) money as compensation (so it's a great idea to hold onto the receipts anyway!). Just remember real jobs come with real fees, so be prepared for the upfront costs as states vary in their license fees. The lowest fee I encountered was $30 (when I applied in Pennsylvania), and the most expensive was $1000 (when I applied in New Jersey).

In order to apply for your license, the state medical boards want to know: Did you graduate medical school? Did you complete a residency? Have you taken/passed boards for your specialty or are you eligible to take the board exam for that specialty?

[1] While that seems simple enough, it becomes more tedious as each of those requirements has multiple proofs of documentation that need to be submitted. Be sure to take a picture of your MD/DO diploma (if given a smaller version, consider scanning onto your computer). For completion of residency training, pictures of your intern year certificate and your residency completion certificate will do (they weren't just wall art for your apartment). You will also need a curriculum vitae (consider having this reviewed by a mentor at your residency so it is formatted correctly) and a board eligibility letter as you will most likely be applying for jobs prior to taking the Pediatric Boards. The board eligibility letter can be usually obtained online from the American Board of Pediatrics website/portal. Once you have these documents, you can start the process! Some of the systems require that this info be input online manually, and some may allow scanned documents for upload.

Some states accept a universal application, which is a system where you upload all necessary documents, complete one application, and then you can submit this application to multiple states. A helpful reference by state for the universal application can be found here [2]:

www.fsmb.org/uniform-application/ua-participating-boards

I discussed earlier the importance of starting this process as soon as you have signed your contract, because there are some states where the process can take up to 6 months for completion. So starting as soon as you find the job or at least at the start of the year can help decrease the risk of any lost time between completion of residency and starting your employment.

Don't feel like you have to have all of this memorized; most state systems online will have a checklist that gets completed along the way to help you keep track of the things left on your to-do list. Lastly, don't forget to select a trustworthy mailing address to ensure that you will receive your license when everything is approved!

DEA/CDS

You got the ok to practice, now you need that thing that allows you to write all of those prescriptions unrestricted!

For physicians there is a nonrefundable fee to obtain your Drug Enforcement Administration (DEA) number, and when I last renewed in 2019, it was $731. You will pay the fee every 3 years (whew a sigh of relief for your wallet!). Additionally, in some states, you are required to also obtain a Controlled Dangerous Substance (CDS) license which allows you to write specifically for controlled substances (e.g., ADHD medications). This CDS is an additional fee (varies by state). To apply for your DEA, log on to the website (with the address and information of the location where you will practice), enter your medical license number, submit the application, and wait. To apply for the CDS, you similarly log on to the website (with your medical license and DEA) and complete the application which may also vary by state (i.e., in NJ there was a paper application which could be accessed via the website, which I completed and mailed in with a $40 check).

Credentialing/Accreditation

Alright! Now we can write notes solo, and write all prescriptions freely! What's next? Getting the actual "privileges/credentials" which will allow you to practice in your office setting is a good next step. This is where your residency coordinator is going to come in handy! As with starting any new chapter, your new employer will want to review your prior track record. Along with all the documents required to obtain your license, your new employer will also wish to have copies of your Basic Life Support and Pediatric Advanced Life Support (BLS/PALS) certifications, your properly formatted CV, your Medicaid provider number (ask your residency coordinator if you don't already know it), National Provider Identifier (NPI, can be googled), and copies of your malpractice insurance coverage throughout residency. Some of my residency colleagues utilized a document service to ease the credentialing process. For this service, you pay a fee and submit all of your documents to a centralized system that allows them to easily just be distributed to your employers for credentialing purposes. This could be beneficial if you have to be credentialed at multiple facilities, or you have to change jobs/career paths. In the interest of being economical, I did not go this route. I took pictures of all the documents and placed them in a folder entitled credentialing documents, to be accessed in the future.

Along with accessing the privileges to work at your new job, you also need to know what type of procedures/skills for which you will be applying. You can determine this easily by emailing your director or discussing with your future colleagues. You may be required to, or wish to, continue to perform procedures such as lumbar punctures, etc. Therefore, this is also a good time to reach out to your residency coordinator to have a copy of your procedure logs and any supporting documentation showing that you are trained for the procedural privileges you are requesting.

Once you have that, as they say "that's all folks!" Now that all of the necessary boring stuff is completed, you are free to focus on the more exciting things, like white coat decor and office plants!

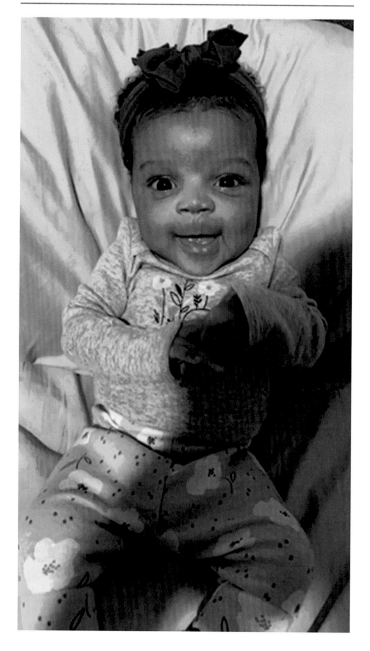

References

1. Obtaining a medical license. American Medical Association, 15 May 2018. www.ama-assn.org/residents-students/career-planning-resource/obtaining-medical-license.
2. UA Participating Boards. Federation of State Medical Boards, 2018. www.fsmb.org/uniform-application/ua-participating-boards/.

Setting Up Your Office

25

Ellen C. Miele

Introduction

What does a pediatric office need? The list can actually be quite short: exam rooms, a waiting and reception area, bathroom facilities, workspace, and a break area. Unlike some other specialties, we don't need a lot of expensive equipment. But there's more to setting up an office than just the space and equipment. If you are starting a practice from scratch, you should consider using a start-up consultant to help you navigate the process. Do your homework! Check out the neighborhoods and local areas. Assess the public transportation. Try to talk to other physicians in both established and newer practices in the area. As you build your physical setup, you need to formulate your office policies as well. For that, you don't need to reinvent the wheel—utilize one of the many online resources to guide you in creating office policies.

Exam Rooms

A good rule of thumb for most busy pediatric practices is three exam rooms per doctor—one room for the patient you are currently seeing, one for the patient you will see next (we all know it can take

E. C. Miele (✉)
Spring Lake Pediatrics, Spring Lake, NJ, USA

© The Author(s), under exclusive license to Springer Nature
Switzerland AG 2021
P. M. Garrett, K. Yoon-Flannery (eds.), *A Pediatrician's Path*,
https://doi.org/10.1007/978-3-030-75370-2_25

a few minutes for parents to get a baby out of the car seat carrier and undressed), and one for the patient you saw last (who is redressing the baby and getting them back into the carrier). Early on you may not have that kind of space, and you may find yourself in a situation where there isn't always a full room for you. You can use the time in between patients to finish charting, make phone calls, or take a quick break. Offering virtual visits that alternate time slots with in-person visits is another way to maximize time and keep the flow of patients moving steadily with fewer exam rooms.

As for furnishings, each exam room should have an exam table for the patient and a seat for the adult who is accompanying them. All exam rooms should also have a sink for handwashing—parents appreciate seeing the doctor wash their hands in the room prior to examining the child. Every exam room should also have a doctor's stool so that you can take a moment at the beginning of every visit and sit while taking the history. Patients' perception of the time spent with a physician is improved when the physician sits down [1].

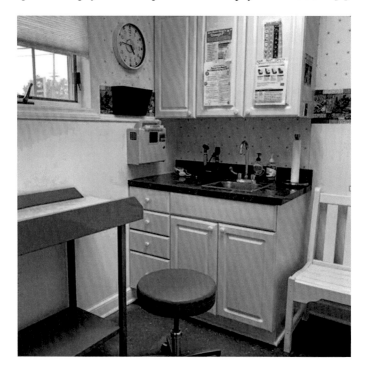

My favorite exam room

Waiting Area and Reception

First, a word about the "waiting" room; proper scheduling is critical to running a practice. Patients should not spend any more than a few minutes in your waiting area. If you routinely have families waiting for 20 minutes or more, then you need to reassess how your scheduling is done.

The COVID-19 pandemic has changed the way doctors use their waiting rooms. Toys and books are gone, and many offices now use the strategy of having patients check-in from their cars. Parents can call or text when they arrive and be called to come into the office once an exam room is open. In areas where patients use public transportation, this isn't feasible, so the waiting room area will be utilized more frequently. Make sure that any and all frequently touched surfaces can be disinfected easily and quickly.

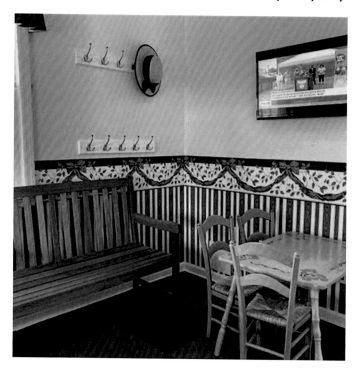

A corner of the waiting room

Always remember that this space is the first impression families get when they enter your office. A friendly receptionist and a welcoming waiting area set the tone for the entire visit. The decor should be inviting and kid friendly with durable furnishings that are easily cleaned but not so juvenile as to make your teenage patients feel out of place. If the area must be carpeted, use carpet tiles/squares to allow for easy replacement when the inevitable spills, pukes, and diaper overflows happen.

Workspace

The physicians and staff need ample space to work on charting and do paperwork. Most offices will also have an area designated as a sort of lab—an area with a sink and enough countertop to allow sufficient room for things like running strep tests and checking urine specimens. The office workspace also needs a refrigerator/freezer for vaccine storage. Proper temperature control is critical for vaccine storage so do not skimp on your fridge! At any given time, you may have tens of thousands of dollars worth of vaccine inventory in your refrigerator, so make it a good one.

Bathrooms

Like the book says, "Everyone Poops." Access to a bathroom is necessary. Ideally, you should have one facility designated for staff and one designated for patients.

Break Area

Doctors and staff need a place to take a break and grab a cup of coffee or sit and eat their lunch. The break area should have comfortable seating, a table, and access to a sink. A small refrigerator and a microwave are nice to have as well. *Food items should never be stored in the same refrigerator as vaccines.*

Decide what perks you want for your staff. A stocked coffee area is a relatively inexpensive gesture that can go a long way toward keeping staff happy. The break area can even be outfitted with space for employees' children for times when childcare is an issue.

Equipment

As long as you have a stethoscope, an ophthalmoscope and otoscope, and appropriately sized blood pressure cuffs, you can perform a comprehensive physical exam. Since our patients can range from 4 pounds to 400 pounds, you will need the ability to weigh and measure patients of all sizes. An infant scale and a regular standing scale are both necessities, as is having a means of measuring patient heights.

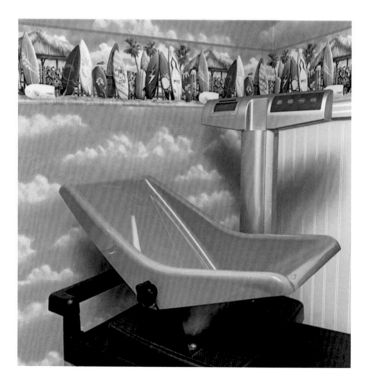

My favorite scale for squirmy kids

Policies

Establishing clear office policies right from the start will assure that every employee knows your expectations and understands their responsibilities from the first day on the job. There are many online resources to help with formulating a comprehensive employee handbook. The AAP offers a sample employee handbook that can be found in the Professional Resources section of the AAP website along with advice on just about every aspect of running an office [2]. All employees must have HIPAA training and should sign an acknowledgment confirming that they have read and understand HIPAA policies.

Infection control policies are another important element that all employees must understand and follow. The CDC's "Guide to Infection Prevention For Outpatient Settings" is an excellent resource for both physicians and staff [3].

Lastly, as your practice grows and becomes successful, you may want to expand. It's never a bad idea to plan for that likelihood right from the start! Choose your location and space wisely so that expansion is less complicated, and make certain that the policies you create are suitable for 2 employees or 20.

References

1. Merel S, McKinney C, Ufkes P, Kwan A, White. A sitting at patients' bedsides may improve patients' perceptions of physician communication skills. J Hosp Med. 2016;11(12):865–8.
2. https://www.aap.org/en-us/professional-resources
3. https://www.cdc.gov/infectioncontrol/pdf/outpatient/guide.pdf

Risk Management and Patient Safety

26

Ursula S. Nawab and Dominic Adams

The Biggest Risk Is Not Talking to Risk

At 5:30 AM, your alarm sounds. You awaken with a smile, realizing that this is the day you've dreamed about for a very long time. Yes, today is your first scheduled shift without supervision. Congratulations! You are now an attending physician. You've put in countless hours in undergraduate school, medical school, and residency, and at last, you've completed your fellowship training. Now is the time for you to bask in the glory of your achievement! Quickly, your brain starts to race. You want to arrive on time for your first shift, ready to get handoff from the departing clinical team. You rush off to shower, get dressed, grab a cup of coffee, and head out the door to begin your commute to work. As you arrive at the medical facility, you look at the surrounding area and take a deep breath. Finally, the moment you've been preparing for is here.

U. S. Nawab (✉)
Perelman School of Medicine, Children's Hospital of Philadelphia, Philadelphia, PA, USA
e-mail: nawabu@chop.edu

D. Adams
Children's Hospitals of Philadelphia, Philadelphia, PA, USA
e-mail: Adamsd1@chop.edu

© The Author(s), under exclusive license to Springer Nature Switzerland AG 2021
P. M. Garrett, K. Yoon-Flannery (eds.), *A Pediatrician's Path*,
https://doi.org/10.1007/978-3-030-75370-2_26

177

As you walk through the doors, you are stopped by Security and informed that you forgot to complete a step in your onboarding process prior to the start of your first day. You inquire about the step you missed. "What step did I not complete?" you ask. The security guard replies, "You forgot to meet with your Risk Manager prior to your official start date." "What is a Risk Manager?" you say.

Of course, this is not what really happens on your first day of work as an attending physician, but it is certainly something that *should* happen. Proactively meeting with a risk manager is a step in the onboarding process that could help you prepare for challenging situations, especially when caring for a patient results in an unexpected outcome.

Getting to know your facility risk manager is one of the most important tasks that you should complete as you begin your new role. Why is meeting with risk management such an important step? The answer is simple – *support*. Risk managers can tell you that after countless interactions between themselves and physicians, a common response from physicians is, "I wish I would have reached out to you sooner for advice and guidance." Support from the risk manager when there's been an unanticipated outcome during patient care can provide you with a mechanism to discuss what should come next. Physicians work endless hours trying to perfect the art of medicine while developing a highly skilled practice. However, it appears that even after all of the medical skills training, creating an equally skillful art in communicating with patients and families remains challenging for many physicians. This is especially true for those physicians who are taking on their first role as an attending physician.

So, what does a meeting with a risk manager entail? First, let's go on record and say the meeting with the risk manager as part of your onboarding process is priceless. During this meeting, the risk manager will define risk management, the role of the risk manager, and the importance of safety event reporting. The risk manager can define and clarify your institution's policies regarding informed consent and advanced directives and discuss the importance of factual, timely, and concise documentation. Risk managers can offer guidance about communicating with challenging patients and families, and they can discuss the importance of disclosure. An understanding of these topics can help you set the foundation for providing safe quality care.

The risk manager will become one of your most important partners in caring for patients. When things go wrong, they will listen, listen again, and do more listening. When you're finally done speaking, the risk manager will ask you how the patient is doing, for your perspective about why/how the event happened, and if the event was disclosed to the patient/family. Then the risk manager will ask you how you're doing, and what support or resources you may need to help you return to providing safe care. Post-event the risk manager will follow up with you to ensure that you have all of the resources you need.

Risk managers are trained to understand the litigious landscape of the healthcare environment. Most have developed skills for identifying when events of harm will likely become a lawsuit. When this happens, if you are named as a defendant in a lawsuit, the risk manager will remain in contact with you regarding the event for the duration of the lawsuit, so that you can feel supported as you continue to provide care to the rest of your patients.

Risk managers understand that there are risks for physicians associated with providing patient care. However, they understand *better* that caring for patients and achieving high-quality outcomes are worth the risk. The risk mitigation strategies, education, and partnership that risk managers will provide to you can help you to deliver excellent patient care with optimal outcomes.

The healthcare industry is very litigious. If you are a named defendant in a lawsuit, please follow these steps to help you throughout the process:

1. Remain cool and partner with your risk management and legal teams to discuss next steps in the process.
2. Be very cooperative with counsel who is assigned to represent you during the duration of the lawsuit. Please be very responsive to emails and phone calls from your assigned attorney.
3. Remember the medical record is your #1 defense in litigation. This should serve as a reminder to document information in the medical record that led to clinical decision-making.

4. A lawsuit is a private matter. Please refrain from discussing the lawsuit outside of authorized personnel assigned to you by the risk and legal department. Text messages, emails, and social media posts are discoverable items in the court of law.

5. Do not take the situation lightly. Always be prepared for depositions. **Never** take call the night before a deposition. **Never** work while on trial.

6. If you are feeling stressed or anxious at any time during the duration of the lawsuit, do not hesitate to contact your risk management or legal team so that they assist with getting you the appropriate resources to support you.

"First Do No Harm" to "To Err Is Human"

After your first day introduction to your risk manager and spending time familiarizing yourself with the electronic health record, you begin to feel comfortable practicing in the "real world" of medicine. Settling in to your workflow and getting to know your patients and the hospital family, your transition has been exciting and rewarding.

One day, on a busy hospital shift with the census at max capacity, the admissions keep coming. As you navigate through the admission orders with three other admissions waiting in the ED, you choose to bypass the medication reconciliation process. Entering the medications manually is simply quicker. While you are putting in the order, your pager goes off, and the nurse informs you that your other patient is desaturating. You get to the bedside quickly after entering 100 mg instead of 10 mg of a benzodiazepine. There was no alert, and you signed the orders. Twenty minutes later, your most recent admission has a code on the floor. The code team arrives and starts CPR. As you are reviewing the record preparing for transfer, you recognize the error and order flumazenil as a reversal agent. The patient is transferred to the ICU.

You did not come to work that day to make a mistake. You did not intend to harm someone. In fact, you discovered the error and reported it to risk and the patient safety teams. Over the next couple of weeks, the patient safety team gets your perspective about the event. During the review, it is noted that the high-dose alert did not fire because it was programmed incorrectly. Instead of being reprimanded, you were asked to be a part of the analysis. Pointing out how the medication reconciliation process was cumbersome, you gave recommendations of how to make it easier to complete. In addition, the human factors team made recommendations to prevent miskeyed values. These changes were made, and the hospital did not have another tenfold overdose medication error, and medication reconciliation was consistently performed throughout the hospital.

In 1999, the Institute of Medicine (IOM) wrote the startling report "To Err Is Human," which acknowledged medical errors and called for development of policies to prevent them. After this seminal paper, patient safety quickly became an important attribute of our healthcare system. At that time, the IOM simply defined patient safety as "freedom from accidental injury." However, as safety science evolved, it was clear that safety is directly related to the system in which care is delivered [3]. The National Patient Safety Foundation took the definition one step further, calling it "avoidance, prevention, and amelioration of adverse outcomes or injuries stemming from the process of care" [3].

Patient safety remains an emerging discipline within the realm of healthcare quality. The science of safety has foundations from fields outside of healthcare, primarily, human factors engineering, system thinking, design thinking, organizational management, and cognitive psychology [3]. The concepts and methodologies are rooted in high-risk industries, such as aviation and nuclear energy.

A safety culture relies on three central attributes: trust, reporting, and learning [9]. Creating a just culture is a critical component of developing a safety culture. An environment of trust is the basis of developing an informed culture [9]. A strong reporting culture relies on psychological safety, organizational behavior, and leader inclusiveness [6]. Nonpunitive response to errors, a feature of psychological safety, fosters an environment in which people feel comfortable to speak up and report [2]. After reporting, a system-based analysis with attention to the operational hazards of the system allows for learning and continuous improvement [9]. Principles of high reliability utilized in other high-risk industries are the fundamental underpinnings of patient safety. These five characteristics of high reliability are [1]:

1. Preoccupation with failure
2. Reluctance to simplify
3. Sensitivity to operations
4. Commitment to resilience
5. Deference to expertise

These principles coupled with a robust safety culture are required to minimize adverse events and eliminate preventable harm.

Even with an active safety culture, adverse events and harm will occur. As long as there is a human in the process, human error happens. The system of care is established by culture, policy and procedures, technology, and education and is designed to provide barriers and checkpoints in healthcare delivery. The healthcare team, however, is the last line of defense. Holes in each layer of the system represent the failures in the barriers put in place to mitigate harm. This is how an adverse event occurs based on Reason's Swiss cheese model [10, 11].

When an event occurs, actions are taken immediately to alleviate any further harm to the patient and disclose the situation. At this point, a systematic evaluation, root cause analysis (RCA), ensues. The RCA is the application of techniques and methodologies to identify the vulnerabilities within the system and to determine system-based improvements. Strong actions as a result of the RCA change the system in a fundamental way, making it easier to do the right thing.

After an unexpected incident resulting from an error occurs, clinicians can be at high risk of experiencing trauma [8]. The associated distress can cause personal, emotional, and even professional problems. This is known as the "second-victim" phenomenon. Feelings of guilt, pain, and isolation can lead to job-related stress and anxiety which can lead to burnout and depression [8]. A strong, supportive, nonpunitive safety culture is associated with increased support for clinicians which can ease or prevent the second-victim trauma [8]. The first tier of support can occur at the local level – event recognition and response training. The next tier of trained peer support is available for an "emotional" debrief (not focusing on the medical care), one-on-one support, and resource identification. The third tier of care involves facilitated referral for ongoing support.

Restorative just culture is a way of approaching safety "differently." This is a concept of replacing hurt with healing. Instead of asking questions of who did what? It asks the questions such as the following: who is hurt; what do they need; and whose obligation is it to meet those needs? [5]. Collaborative resolution of these questions can lead to forward-thinking results by answering the questions of "who needs to do what now." The goal being engagement, emotional healing, and reintegration of those involved combined with organizational learning and improvement, understanding what "went wrong and why" when there is an undesirable outcome is safety I. This is the reactive arm of safety and is helpful in understanding rare but catastrophic events. Knowing "what went right" is safety II. This is important to recognize, as this applies to the majority of health care. Improving healthcare safety requires both arms of safety. Focusing solely on safety I can result in rigid processes and increased constraints, straining the complex adaptive system of health care [7]. Safety II asserts that variations in work, in order to adapt to the increased complexities of health care, contribute to optimal outcomes (Table 26.1). Resilience and adaptive capacity are utilized by individuals and systems in response to unanticipated threats thus contributing to institutional learning [7]. Relying primarily on safety II contributes to habituation which leads to underappreciation of safety risk. By understanding why things happen (the good and the bad), we can learn and continually improve the care we give to our patients, ourselves, and our colleagues.

Table 26.1 Overview of safety I and safety II

	Safety I	Safety II
Definition of safety	That as few things as possible go wrong	That as many things as possible go right
Safety management principle	Reactive, respond when something happens or is categorized as an unacceptable risk	Proactive, continuously trying to anticipate developments and events
View of the human factor in safety management	Humans are predominantly seen as a liability or hazard. They are a problem to be fixed	Humans are seen as a resource necessary for system flexibility and resilience. They provide flexible solutions to many potential problems
Accident investigation	Accidents are caused by failures and malfunctions. The purpose of an investigation is to identify the causes	Things basically happen in the same way, regardless of the outcome. The purpose of an investigation is to understand how things usually go right as a basis for explaining how things occasionally go wrong
Risk assessment	Accidents are caused by failures and malfunctions. The purpose of an investigation is to identify causes and contributory factors	To understand the conditions where performance variability can become difficult or impossible to monitor and control

Source: Hollnagel [4]

References

1. Cochrane BS, Hagins MJ, Picciano G, King JA, Marshall DA, Nelson B, Deao C. High reliability in healthcare: creating the culture and mindset for patient safety. Healthc Manage Forum. 2017;30(2):61–8. https://doi.org/10.1177/0840470416689314.
2. Edmondson AC. The fearless organization. Hoboken: John Wiley & Sons, Ltd.; 2019.
3. Emanuel L, Berwick D, Conway J, Combes J, Hatlie M, Leape L, et al. (2008) What exactly is patient safety? In K. Henriksen, J. B. Battles, M. A. Keyes, & M. L. Grady (Eds.). Rockville.
4. Hollnagel E, Wears RL, Braithwaite J (2015) From safety-I to safety-II: a white paper. The Resilient Health Care Net: Published simultaneously by

the University of Southern Denmark, University of Florida, USA, and Macquarie University, Australia.

5. Kaur M, de Boer R, Oates A, Rafferty J, Dekker S. Restorative just culture: a study of the practical and economic effects of implementing restorative justice in an NHS trust. MATEC Web of Conferences. 2019;273:1007. https://doi.org/10.1051/matecconf/201927301007.

6. Nembhard I, Edmondson A. Making it safe: the effects of leader inclusiveness and professional status on psychological safety and improvement efforts in health care teams. J Organ Behav. 2006;27:941–66. https://doi.org/10.1002/job.413.

7. Patterson M, Deutsch ES. Safety-I, safety-II and resilience engineering. Curr Probl Pediatr Adolesc Health Care. 2015;45(12):382–9. https://doi.org/10.1016/j.cppeds.2015.10.001.

8. Quillivan RR, Burlison JD, Browne EK, Scott SD, Hoffman JM. Patient safety culture and the second victim phenomenon: connecting culture to staff distress in nurses. Jt Comm J Qual Patient Saf. 2016;42(8):377–86. https://doi.org/10.1016/s1553-7250(16)42053-2.

9. Reason J, Hobbs A. Managing maintenance error: a practical guide. Boca Raton: CRC Press; 2003.

10. Reason JT. Human error. Cambridge [England]; New York: Cambridge University Press; 1990.

11. Seshia SS, Bryan Young G, Makhinson M, Smith PA, Stobart K, Croskerry P. Gating the holes in the Swiss cheese (part I): expanding professor Reason's model for patient safety. J Eval Clin Pract. 2018;24(1):187–97. https://doi.org/10.1111/jep.12847.

Mentorship

27

Joannie Yeh

The Origin of Mentorship

Mentorship accelerates personal and professional growth. While residency may have offered easy access to official and informal opportunities for mentorship, intentional networking after graduation can continue to provide a source for valuable mentor relationships. This chapter will outline how to seek and cultivate productive mentorships as a mentee, but first, a brief flashback to a classic story by Homer.

The character Mentor is commonly brought up in mentorship discussions because he is an old family friend who advises Telemachus, the son of Odysseus, while Odysseus is away. He is often seen to embody the traits of experience and trust, which is the basis of the Dictionary.com definition of a mentor as "an experienced and a trusted advisor." However, Mentor only succeeded in guiding the clueless Telemachus after Athena appeared in his form [1]. Yes, the true hero and mentor was not Mentor, but rather Athena, the Greek goddess of wisdom.

J. Yeh (✉)
Sidney Kimmel Medical College, Philadelphia, PA, USA;
https://www.betamomma.com

© The Author(s), under exclusive license to Springer Nature Switzerland AG 2021
P. M. Garrett, K. Yoon-Flannery (eds.), *A Pediatrician's Path*,
https://doi.org/10.1007/978-3-030-75370-2_27

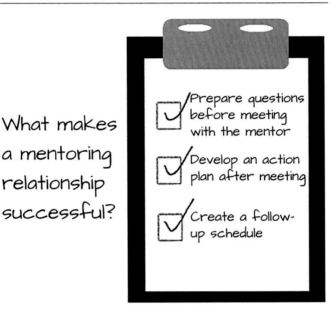

Find Yourself Before Finding a Mentor

Now, throw that story out and let's rewrite it with you, the mentee, as the hero. First, as a residency graduate, you are a lot more motivated and skilled at problem-solving than Telemachus. Our starting point is a lot further than where the helpless Telemachus was. We are capable of meeting our mentor halfway. Believe in the accomplishments and experiences you have already acquired. They are a strong enough foundation upon which to continue building your career and life.

- What have you already done?
- In which direction would you like to take your career?
- What questions, struggles, or gaps do you foresee in reaching your career goals?

Knowing your own interests and strengths can help you find a fitting mentor. Look for someone who is already in a position in which you would like to see yourself in the future. It doesn't have to be an exact clone of "future you," just some part of "future you." If you would like to be a private practice physician who works with a global health organization and teaches medical students, then a potential mentor might match one or two of those categories.

Where to Find a Mentor

As a residency graduate in this modern life, there is no Athena. There may be no perfect mentor. While we probably don't have the luck of happening upon a Greek goddess who takes an interest in us and swoops into our life to coach us into empowerment, we don't need luck. We just need to look. We can start by looking in the hospital for familiar attendings, research investigators, and department chairs. We can also look at Facebook groups, Twitter, LinkedIn, and hospital websites for potential mentors (see the *Social Media* chapter). We can look through a Google search.

Invite other people to help you find a mentor. Share your interest in looking for a mentor with peers, prior mentors and attendings, and friends on social media platforms. Someone will always know someone who can help you. You don't have Athena, but you have Google and networking. Have you tried this yet? If not, take 10 minutes today to reach out to three people. They can be a potential mentor within your network, a friend or acquaintance that might know a potential mentor, or someone you found from Google. Send three e-mails. (Not sure what your interests are yet? Take 10 minutes to brainstorm about that and call a friend to talk about it.) You will find your mentor.

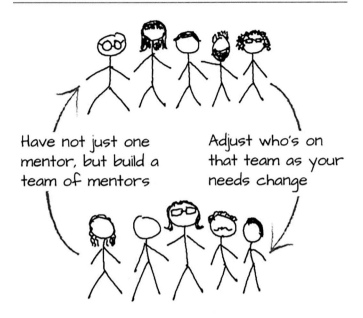

Now, in lieu of Athena, who is a multitalented goddess of many things, keep in mind that you can have not just one, but many mentors. It's okay to reevaluate your mentor relationship at a later time and reconsider if it is still beneficial for you. Perhaps you are looking for growth in a new skill or in a role that is not familiar to your current mentor. Perhaps your mentor is overscheduled and is no longer as responsive to requests for meetings or to answering e-mails. In that case, look for a new mentor. Needs and situations change. It's okay to change mentors, too. Instead of access to a goddess mentor, collect a village of mentors.

Making the Most of the Mentoring Relationships

As with being intentional in finding a mentor, also be intentional in how you spend time with your mentor. Be prepared with an agenda and with questions you have. Provide an update on your progress and what you plan your next steps to be. Be transparent about where you are struggling to meet your goals. This gives purpose to the meeting (and always ask yourself first if a meeting is necessary) and direction to the discussions.

After your meetings, send an e-mail with a brief summary of ideas you discussed as well as a list of your action items and a timeline for completing them. Then, schedule a date to send a follow-up e-mail to your mentor to let them know where you are in the process and if you have any further questions. This helps keep you accountable. Don't rely on your busy mentor to check in – although this is wonderful if they can do that, too. By initiating those e-mails, you can take control of making progress and making the most out of mentoring relationships.

Summary
1. Brainstorm and know your career goals.
2. Find a mentor who can help you reach those goals.
3. Find additional mentors as needed.
4. Create an agenda for your meetings.
5. Make your own action items.
6. Schedule follow up meetings with your mentor.

Reference

1. O'Donnell BRG. (October 13, 2017). *The Odyssey*'s millennia-old model of mentorship. *The Atlantic*. https://www.theatlantic.com/business/archive/2017/10/the-odyssey-mentorship/542676/.

The Patient Experience

Tanushree Singhal

Introduction

As we are talking about patient experience, I am going to assume that you have finished your training and are heading towards the next milestone, be it a new job at a private practice, in a hospital-based larger practice, or maybe you are starting your own practice.

So you have completed your training and you have landed a dream job. All is good now. You can sit back and relax. See patients 8 am to 5 pm and you are done…correct? Not really.

Because now that you have entered the real world, you are an attending physician and are in charge of decision-making. These decisions impact you and your patients' lives. These are not easy decisions. With these decisions and how you convey them, you form bonds with patients and their families. These bonds are the backbone of the patient experience.

During medical school and residency, emphasis is on learning, managing sick people, and delivering health care. But in the real world, another important component is the patient experience.

T. Singhal (✉)
Department of Pediatrics, Mayo Clinic Health System,
EAU CLAIRE, WI, USA

© The Author(s), under exclusive license to Springer Nature
Switzerland AG 2021
P. M. Garrett, K. Yoon-Flannery (eds.), *A Pediatrician's Path*,
https://doi.org/10.1007/978-3-030-75370-2_28

Unless your patients trust you, they are not likely to be compliant. They are not likely to come back to you. Not just you but the entire system relies on patient experience for efficient delivery of health care. Whether you are an outpatient clinician or a hospitalist, whether you work in a small rural setting or large hospital owned practice, patient experience matters to all. Hence, institutions are investing millions in this field and hiring employees to focus on "patient experience." There are several tools available to measure patient experience, including Avatar, Press Ganey, and others.

For a fresh-out-of-training new hire, what should be your focus? Of course you have made sure your contract is bona fide, you have good malpractice coverage, you are stepping into a welcoming practice with good co-workers and staff, and your pay is good.

Now that you have started seeing patients and are enjoying your work, you have had some good interactions with patients. Imagine that one day you receive a letter saying "I felt Dr S was rushed through the appointment. She arrived 10 minutes late and my child was out of control by then as it was his nap time." You certainly didn't expect this. You thought you had a positive interaction, but the patient (or parent) didn't think so. You are left disheartened and feel very low. Then you start analyzing. You go through your schedule that day and recall that the patient before that presented for one small concern, but as you started asking questions, their complaint became much bigger. You were not able to complete this visit in your allotted 20 minutes and did go into your next appointment late. Then you start thinking about your own children and their nap times and how cranky they get when they don't nap on time. And then you realize that the patient was right.

So how do you resolve this situation? You can call the family if your practice is okay with it (most practices actually encourage this), apologize, and explain what happened. Believe me one small step will go a long way toward improving your relationship with your patients and building trust. Learn to apologize early on. There will be times when your patient or parent will be grumpy from an already terrible home situation or illness and then may not enjoy the check in process and interaction with staff. If you show your empathy about how their day has been and say something like "let us try and make most out of this appointment and help Johnny feel better," you may already be at an advantage with them.

With technical advances, everyone is looking at numbers, data, and graphs. Medicine is all about these. But remember when you entered this field, you had a purpose to treat children; never forget your purpose, and never forget your human touch. Any successful doctor first has that connection with his patients. Always take your time and try making eye contact and not looking at the screen when addressing your patient's concerns. A warm, caring bedside manner will go a long way to establish positive patient relations. Some practices even hire specialists to give advice on facilitating patient relations. They will guide you and give tools to help you improve.

About Vendors

If you are going into private practice or starting your own practice, it is important to know a little about the vendors and the cost of surveying patients. There are several vendors out there; Professional Research Consultant (PRC), Press Ganey, and Avatar are some of the more commonly used companies. PRC is considered one of the best but it is also one of the most costly. They perform telephonic surveys so are more likely to get a response. Since they rely on manpower, it is expensive. There are several vendors that send out paper surveys. Because these also have to be scored manually, they can be costly as well. Email surveys are the cheapest. There are several free tools you can use; one of them is Survey Monkey. For physicians who see patients with Medicaid insurance, there is a Medicaid survey which helps in improving your reimbursement. In order to utilize this feature, you do have to show an ongoing relationship with your patient for at least 6 months. It is important to make sure whichever survey you are using is HIPAA compliant. Also remember the purpose of collecting this data is to show improvement, not to see who is "the best."

My institution uses Press Ganey, a very popular vendor for surveying patients. As it is a large institution, with thousands of doctors and advanced practice providers (APPs), thousands of surveys are sent out, and millions of dollars are spent on this endeavor.

Why Do This?

It is mandatory for Magnet certification, the Joint Commission, inpatient services, and dialysis. There are also the US Department of Health and Human Services and Centers for Medicare and Medicaid requirements.

There is an inpatient behavioral health requirement.

You are doing this to get feedback so you can improve on your practice.

Your payers and insurance companies want you to do them.

Additionally, this is not something you can do once and be done with; it is a continuous work in progress. Once you reach a certain benchmark, you have to keep going up. It is a never ending race.

Press Ganey Scoring/Analyzing

MDs and APPs get a score based on the survey, which is a 5 point scale. A 5 is considered good, and a 1 is considered poor. Most doctors have an average score of 4 or 5. There is also a percentile score which is a comparison at the national level based on surveys of hospitals all over the country. The questions that are generally asked on a Press Ganey survey include:

- Concern the care provider showed for your questions or worries
- Explanations the care provider gave you about your problem or condition
- Care provider's efforts to include you in decisions about your treatment
- Degree to which care provider talked with you using words you could understand

- Amount of time the care provider spent with you
- Friendliness/courtesy of the care provider
- Information the care provider gave you about medications (if any)
- Your confidence in this care provider
- Likelihood of your recommending this care provider to others
- Instructions the care provider gave you about follow-up care (if any)

A survey is definitely not all-encompassing, but it is a way to capture a snapshot of care.

For us in pediatrics, there are several concerns. First, we are not surveying our patients but their parents and guardians. There may be custody issues, or privacy concerns with teenagers. Also, the return rate for surveys is lower. In pediatric subspecialties, scores may be lower because there are less patients seen when compared to primary care, and thus a lower number of surveys conducted. One low score will have a greater impact in this situation.

I read this on kauferdmc.com, a marketing website and that seems to resonate here:

> Happy customers are typically open to the idea of writing a review. Unhappy customers, on the other hand, are motivated to write a negative review. But both are in the minority.

Outcome/Grievance

To give you an overview of what happens at ground level in bigger practices, once a grievance is received, it is recorded and tracked until there is a closure. An email is sent to the leaders including the chairperson of the department, and the provider in question is also asked to give their input. Once a response is received, a letter is drafted and sent to the patient for closure. For any financial adjustment, there is a reviewing committee that decides if there will be a payout. If it involves more than $500 (or so), there is a reviewing team that determines how much the payment will be.

Once a grievance is received, it has to be resolved within 7 days as per the Joint Commission. If it cannot be resolved in 7 days, then an acknowledgement letter should be sent to the patient. This gives the institution an extra 30 days to review and respond back. There is a letter sent every 30 days until a closure is achieved.

Below is one of my favorite tools, called PEARLS, from Academy of Communications in Healthcare (ACH). It is a technique designed to create trust and build rapport with patients, and hopefully it will help you increase your patient experience scores!

- *Partnership* – Using "we" and "us" promotes shared decision-making.
- *Empathy* – Responding compassionately to the facts and emotions of a patient's situation.
- *Apology* – Expressing regret when you are wrong or in error. It can reduce strong emotion and must be authentic to be effective.
- *Respect* – Showing that you value the patient's decisions and have disciplined yourself to become aware of unconscious bias.
- *Legitimization* – Validation of patient's concerns, feelings, and choices. It does not require agreement and helps move the conversation beyond an impasse.
- *Support* – Assess the patient's level of support and explain how you will support their care. "I am here for you."

Suggested Reading

1. Press Ganey. Mayo Clinic patient experience. http://intranet.mayo.edu/charlie/quality/files/2018/03/Provider-Resources-by-Survey-Type-7-10-17.pdf.
2. http://www.pressganey.com/. Press Ganey Corporation, 401 Edgewater Place, Ste 500, Wakefield, MA 01880. Accessed 7 July 2021.
3. https://kauferdmc.com/. 144 Railroad Ave Suite 222 Edmonds, WA 98020. Accessed 7 July 2021.
4. https://www.hopkinsmedicine.org/office-of-johns-hopkins-physicians/best-practice-news/defusing-difficult-situations. Accessed 7 July 2021.

Part IV

After Starting Your First Job

Preparing for Your First Day

29

Kanika Gupta

Welcome to your first day as an attending physician! Your first day as an attending can be a daunting prospect, but it should be an exciting one. Remember that this has been your goal throughout all of medical school, residency, and possibly fellowship. Congratulations, you made it!

Before your first day, most institutions will have made sure that you complete paperwork for onboarding, credentialing, computer training, and safety modules. Pay attention to these as it can give you important insights into the culture of your new workplace and provide you with valuable information that you may need.

The first few days will involve orientation and should involve direct time shadowing other attendings in a similar job role. If this isn't offered, ask for it! During orientation, don't focus as much on the clinical medicine but use this opportunity to observe workflow and get accustomed to how this particular office or hospital runs.

One of the most important and exciting parts of your first day is meeting all of your colleagues – including co-attendings, nurses, administrative staff, MAs, techs, maintenance, residents, students, and everyone else that helps keep everything running smoothly! Even if you are shy or it feels awkward, try to make an

K. Gupta (✉)
Division of General Pediatrics, Nemours Alfred I. duPont Hospital for Children, Wilmington, DE, USA
e-mail: Kanika.gupta@nemours.org

© The Author(s), under exclusive license to Springer Nature Switzerland AG 2021
P. M. Garrett, K. Yoon-Flannery (eds.), *A Pediatrician's Path*,
https://doi.org/10.1007/978-3-030-75370-2_29

effort to introduce yourself and say hello to everyone you meet. Bonus points if you remember their names and roles. First impressions count!

Transitioning from training to an attending position is challenging, and it is important to recognize that it may require a shift in mentality. Your medical journey thus far has often been simply about *surviving training*. You may have told yourself "I just need to get through these four years of medical school, I just need to complete residency, I just need to finish fellowship." You've made it through training, now what?

It is critical that you approach your new attending job with the mindset that it is and will be your forever job. Even if you know that it is only temporary, or you consider your new position as a starter job, or if you're waiting for your partner to finish up training, this definitive shift in your mentality will enrich your experience and make the whole process much more enjoyable. Also, as an attending, connections and professionalism become even more paramount and you never know when connections will become important in the future.

Your first attending job, no matter where it is, is a period of huge growth with an enormous learning curve. Some of this growth is clinically focused – since it is now your medical license in jeopardy, it is only natural to second-guess some decisions that you would have made without thinking during training. Remember that your training has prepared you well clinically. Most of the steep learning curve is more systems-based: learning office procedures, how to reach consultants if you need help, basic phone numbers, and how to navigate the EMR. Your days can now involve prior authorizations, contributing to team meetings, figuring out how much PTO time you want to take, or becoming the lead on clinical or research initiatives. It takes time to figure this out, and you should expect to be less efficient than you are used to in the beginning. Don't worry, things will get easier and faster! Know your limitations and recognize that adjusting to work as an attending requires some time. Enjoy yourself! There is so much that will become part of your daily work routine that isn't taught during training.

Use your orientation period and your first few months on the job to ask lots of questions! It is generally harder to ask questions after you have been at a job for over 6 months, so make sure you take this opportunity to ask lots of questions – no matter how trivial they may seem to you. How do I call the operator? Where do I park? Where are the bathrooms? What should I do if I need immediate assistance with a patient? Remember that your new employer doesn't expect you to know how to perform all parts of your new job! Ask for documents you can refer to that detail clinical pathways, your local-area resources, and important phone numbers. Asking questions helps you and simultaneously also shows you are dedicated to high-performance quality care and that you are dedicated to making this new job sustainable.

Finally, remember that your employer didn't hire you simply for your clinical acumen or how much you have published. Your letters of reference and interviews all were to evaluate your professionalism, attitude, and passion – they were clearly impressed because they hired you! Embrace the self-doubt and keep up this motivation to learn and stay excited!

Daily Considerations

30

Sarah M. Taub

Introduction

Interviewing and finding your first job as an attending physician after residency can be both exciting and frightening. But once you have signed the contract, it is time to start your new educational path as an attending pediatrician. I wanted to focus on a few areas of your new day-to-day life that will help make that transition a little easier.

Scheduling

Part of this journey does require some forethought and attention to the details of your new position. Starting with scheduling, you will need to understand the specific flow of your office. Most offices have schedules in blocks of time allowed for well child visits and sick visits, and most, if not all practices, have EHR that can allow for patients to self-schedule. The time of each visit will vary by office, and understanding if you have flexibility in

S. M. Taub (✉)
Children's Hospital of Philadelphia, Care Network Norristown, Norristown, PA, USA

scheduling is important. For instance, if you are seeing a new patient with multiple medical issues, or a child with behavioral or mental health issues, are you allowed extra time? Getting familiar with this will be key to managing your time during the day.

Patients are usually scheduled in increments of 10–15 minute time slots. Many EHRs are flexible in scheduling patients according to each individual practitioner. In my experience, I have worked in offices which allow only 15 minutes per well child, and then other offices that allow 30 minutes for adolescents or complex children. Sick appointments are usually faster, and some offices schedule them in blocks of 10 minutes. Be aware that you can also be double-booked, which means that you would have more than one patient booked in the same time slot. This could be done during busy winter seasons to add on patients, or if your office has a percentage of patients who do not show for appointments; this is another way to offset that loss of revenue. Some offices also allow for walk-in time, so that patients do not require an appointment and allow patients flexibility to come in when they need to without the barrier of scheduling a time beforehand.

If you have the time and available staff, it is a good practice to huddle in the morning and review the patient list for the day. This will allow you to build in extra time as needed and discuss what the upcoming procedures for the day will look like for you and your staff. While it is not perfect, and problems always arise, I have found this tool to be useful, and it also creates a space that allows your staff to have input and work as a team.

Call Schedule/Hospital Rounds

Being on-call or performing hospital rounds is usually an integrated part of a private practice schedule. Some practices rotate on-call schedules with other group practices, and/or they have either an in-house or outsourced triage phone system. Phone triage can greatly reduce the number of phone calls that you receive and allow you to have a better night's sleep.

Hospital rounds typically occur before office visits, and some practices allow time for going to the hospital(s), while others expect that you make rounds prior to starting regular office hours. The location of the hospital(s) can greatly alter your daily schedule. Usually the hospital rounds are divided among the providers working in the office that week or weekend.

Weekend schedules can vary greatly when you are on-call for that weekend. Some offices offer well visits and sick visits on the weekends and may be open both Saturday and Sunday, and others may only be open on Saturday. Most outpatient offices offer hours on the weekends for their patients. Usually the person working on the weekend will also make hospital rounds for both days of the weekend and take the phone calls. These weekend on-call schedules are usually shared among the providers, and during the busy winter season, you may be working with others. Depending on where you are working, access to emergency rooms and urgent cares may dictate your work schedule. It is also not uncommon to have unequal distribution of this burden — that some of the more senior physicians may work fewer weekends and take less phone calls.

Evening Hours

Most offices need to offer evening appointments to accommodate working families. Practitioners usually work at least one evening per week and may be paired with other providers depending on the size of the group and the need for visits.

Documentation

Almost all private- and hospital-based practices have EHR, and there are many different platforms. If you are not familiar with the EHR that you will be using, then it is imperative that you receive training and spend time getting familiar with the EHR. More than likely, finishing charts may not occur during the work day, especially during the busy winter season. Make sure you can connect to your EHR from home and know what your office policy is for completing charts. Remember, if your colleague were to see your patient the next day, make sure they have enough information to understand your thought process and/or diagnosis (even if you have not completed that visit).

Office Staff

As in residency, you will work very closely with your office staff. You may also be working more or less hours than you did in residency, depending on the schedule of your office. I would advise you to think of the staff (both medical and nonmedical) you worked with in your residency clinic and use those relationships as a sounding board for your new practice. In other words, what qualities in those people that you enjoyed working alongside would you like to see in your future office staff?

One of the most important office staff is the office manager, who usually controls the physician and nurse/MA schedule alongside the lead physicians. This person will be someone that also controls something very dear to you – your vacation time. Take the time to get to know this individual and also ask others how they get along with him/her. Does the staff respect this individual and in turn feel supported by this person? In my experience, I have worked with both effective and ineffective managers, and they both have very different impacts on the office. Even the more effective office manager, while running a smooth operation, often did the bidding of the lead physician and did not support the staff. I would also inquire as to how long that person has held the position, as that will tell you a lot about how the office dynamics work. If office managers are turning over, it is likely a sign of some trouble from leadership or other personality conflicts within the office.

Other office personnel to consider are your support network of either nurses or medical assistants. These will be the staff with whom you work most closely every day. Consider how well they are treated by the other physicians and how well they work together. If the support staff has been working in the office for a long time, that is a great sign that they enjoy working together as a team. If there has been a lot of turnover, that can be a signal that the team is not working well, or there is a disconnect between the leadership (physicians and managers) and support staff. Talk to the office staff as well as the physicians to get a sense of their level of happiness in the workplace. It is also important to know how many nurses/MAs are working alongside the physicians and also if there are additional people answering phones or making appointments. Many offices have to deal with times of being understaffed, but if that is a constant in the workplace, that can place a lot of pressure on physicians and staff and lead to burnout.

The front desk staff is very vital and important to any outpatient practice. They are the first faces and voices that the patients interact with, and often on a regular basis. Do they seem friendly and answer the phone politely? Do they seem to know the patients when they come into the office? As you likely know already, the first person our patients interact with usually sets the tone for the entire visit. Their job can be difficult, as they often bear the brunt of frustrated or anxious parents.

Lastly, another group is the other physicians or advanced practice providers you will be working with. As you may have felt in residency, the team approach always works the best. You need to feel that you share the same views about practice management and schedules. It is also important that your colleagues support one another and will fill in for you when you are sick or need a leave of absence. Work will become a second home, and without a sense of collaboration and willingness to help one another out, it will make the work experience much harder. Oftentimes you have to plan your life 6 months or more ahead of time due to patient scheduling. If you have a good team that is willing to be flexible and help out, then when things come up in life (which they inevitably do), you will feel that you have a team behind you.

Vacations

You will need to take a vacation from time to time, and your co-workers will have to work your hours or accommodate for your absence. And the reverse is true when your colleagues are out of the office. As a result, most practices have to schedule provider vacations well in advance, as patients may need to schedule up to 6 months in advance (or sometimes more). This can be a challenge for you and your family to plan your vacation time so far in advance. Again, having a supportive team behind you can greatly reduce some of this stress.

Leave of Absence

And this leads into where your group stands for the possible leave of absence, either for medical reasons or other. How does your group handle short-term leave? Will your group support your decision to take time off and cover your shifts? Contracts should include policies for short- and long-term leave of absence, and policies will differ among different group practices. While you may not be thinking of this issue at the start of your new position, it will most invariably come up during your career, whether for family planning or medical issues.

Electronic Health Records

31

Adam Glasofer

Electronic health records (EHRs) are made by technical resources, most of whom have never worked a clinical day in their life, and have little to no knowledge of clinical workflows or clinical information. A good EHR vendor will collaborate with clinicians to make sure they approximate the workflow as closely as possible. That being said, no EHR is anywhere close to perfect. They are information systems designed to capture as much structured data as possible, often at the expense of the narrative elements of patient care. This allows EHRs to become valuable tools for healthcare organizations as they can ingest massive amounts of data and provide actionable insights with regard to patient care, operational efficiency, and revenue. They also create an environment where health systems can begin to use next-level computing processes like artificial intelligence and machine learning to provide intelligent, real-time clinical decision support. While these technical advances will no doubt drive medicine into a whole new generation, the role of the EHR has garnered a lot of negative attention for how it has changed the interaction between patient and provider and for contributing to the high rates of provider burnout. In pointing this out, my intention is not to scare you but

A. Glasofer (✉)
Information Technology, Virtua Health, Marlton, NJ, USA
e-mail: aglasofer2@virtua.org

P. M. Garrett, K. Yoon-Flannery (eds.), *A Pediatrician's Path*,
https://doi.org/10.1007/978-3-030-75370-2_31

211

to make you realize that EHRs are not going away. So, best to be aware of some of the issues they may potentially create and address them head on.

Now that we've gotten all of that out of the way, let's look at what type of relationship you may have with the EHR. As the Associate Chief Medical Information Officer (ACMIO) of a large suburban community health system, I am often on the receiving end of comments related to our EHR. What I've learned over time is that, like it or not, a clinician's relationship with the EHR is a critical element in the delivery of care. If you want to make your job easier, embrace this notion and make the EHR work for you, just as you would any other tool in your clinical arsenal (stethoscope, otoscope, etc.).

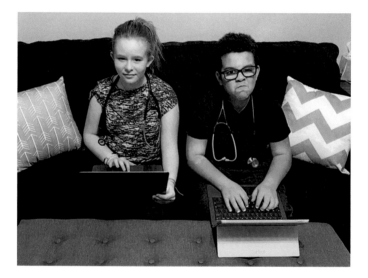

Unsurprisingly, the EHR relationship types are essentially a bell-shaped curve that mimic other types of technology adoption. Here are the three types of relationships you'll see:

1. *Adversarial*

   These providers are typically extremely resistant to change and largely unwilling to adopt anything new, let alone technology. They will often submit, but only while kicking and screaming. Sadly, in doing so, they miss out on many of the advantages an EHR could provide them in maximizing their efficiency. Despite best efforts, they will likely never become open minded enough to do so either. They know how to get their work done in the EHR and that's enough for them. If they had their way, they would likely still be scribbling illegibly on paper.

2. *Accepting*

   These providers are the bulk of the bell curve and accept that change is necessary but often do just enough to get by. Within this spectrum, you'll see a range of behaviors that go from doing the bare minimum to using some advanced EHR tools like voice recognition, macros, and smart texts. The nice thing about this group is that they are often open minded and eager to hear about shortcuts that will make their jobs easier but at the same time will not seek this information out on their own.

3. *Advanced*

   These providers have put in the time to master the system and it shows. They use all potential EHR tools that are available to them in order to maximize their efficiency of documentation and task performance within their given clinical workflow. These are providers that never stay late to document or take charts home with them because they have taken full advantage of integrating the EHR in order to keep as much work as possible at the office or hospital.

As you enter a new job or new health system, I would encourage you to work toward an advanced EHR-type relationship and view the EHR as an important clinical tool that you can use to your benefit. Don't just stop at getting the required training. Instead, seek out training resources to learn advanced tools to streamline your usage, documentation, and task performance. It will take some extra time outside of clinical hours to do this, but the investment will be well worth it. You'll develop skills that will allow you to become more efficient at doing your job than many of your colleagues. And at the end of the day, you'll leave the office or hospital less stressed and likely with little to no EHR work to be done after hours. But like any good lasting relationship, it takes work. Be sure to check in with new EHR education and enhancements every once in a while to make sure you're doing all you can to keep up the success.

Lastly, and perhaps most importantly, document as you go. I cannot stress this enough. What will take 2–3 minutes in real time will take 2–3 times as long later. We are constantly hearing stories of docs spending hours on end after clinical work finishing their EHR work and seeing countless reports about provider burnout due to the EHR. These providers have likely not put in the time to maximize their efficiency but are also likely not documenting in real time. Unless someone has a life-threatening condition, they can wait another couple of minutes so that you can complete all EHR tasks from the patient you just saw. In the over 10 years I've been providing clinical care, I can honestly say that I can count on both hands the number of times I had to stay late for EHR work or bring it home with me. After all, your time is worth something, and I've yet to see a health system pay providers for bringing work home with them.

So in summary, put yourself in a position so that the EHR is working for you and not the other way around. It will take some upfront time commitment, but the amount of time you will save in the long run is immeasurable. And even more importantly, the positive relationship you develop with the EHR by viewing it as a valuable clinical tool will help to keep you from feeling as though you are captive and are instead in control. In doing so, you'll put yourself in the best position possible to avoid burnout and to preserve the patient interactions that likely brought you into medicine in the first place.

Asking for Help

32

Angela Michaels

Introduction

As a student, it wasn't a question of whether to ask for help—the assumption was you would need assistance with even the smallest of tasks and people were prepared for an endless list of questions from you. As a trainee, you probably soaked up every ounce of advice given, although toward the end of your training, it may have come more unsolicited. As a newly independent physician, you will likely feel overwhelmed with responsibility but unsure of when to seek help. Knowing your surroundings, resources, and your own comforts and limits will help you succeed in your role as an attending physician.

Pick a Job That Fits Your Needs

When seriously considering a job, ask yourself what type of environment you would need to feel comfortable. Will you thrive as the only provider covering a rural inpatient ward? Do you feel most at ease with having several other providers in-office to bounce ideas off of? Awareness of your style of practice will help

A. Michaels (✉)
Department of Pediatrics, Division of Neonatal-Perinatal Medicine,
Wake Forest Baptist Health, Winston-Salem, NC, USA

© The Author(s), under exclusive license to Springer Nature
Switzerland AG 2021
P. M. Garrett, K. Yoon-Flannery (eds.), *A Pediatrician's Path*,
https://doi.org/10.1007/978-3-030-75370-2_32

identify a well-matched position. Some early-career physicians may find they are uncomfortable with fewer resources to rely on, whereas others may feel it will help them develop their practice. Regardless, it is helpful to discuss during interviews what the employees do when they have both clinical and institutional questions.

Interviews may or may not include an overview of their orientation process. While questions will always arise, the largest number will occur in those first 3–6 months at a new position. Before accepting a position, set clear expectations of how they will help you acclimate so that you know what to expect.

Get to Know Your Environment

The size and type of practice you entered may heavily influence your resources. A three-person general practice may mean a couple close-knit colleagues who all have a large patient panel, see newborns at the local hospital, and take a third of the nights for after-hours calls. Joining an eight-person subspecialty division might mean more environments to learn—inpatient, procedural, outpatient and consults—but more resources and more well-established guidelines with a structured onboarding process.

You will usually find people who are more enthusiastic about helping others and can ask advice more frequently from them. If you feel that your requests for assistance are not being addressed, identifying someone more formally as your mentor or resource may improve their responsiveness. Especially for clinical advice or to ask about sensitive issues, old mentors such as program directors or colleagues such as co-residents can function as additional sounding boards.

You may also find that you have different colleagues you approach depending on the question, and factors that influence those preferences may be personality-, experience-, and comfort-based. For example, questions about "routine" tasks or basic management practices may be easy to ask any colleague, whereas a rare or complex problem may be best addressed to more experienced co-workers.

Especially with regard to clinical questions, assure you can have a dialogue with whomever you ask. You do not simply want someone to "give you a fish" but rather "teach you how to fish"; aim to obtain not just a suggestion, but the understanding behind it. You will find that some colleagues align more, and others less, with your management style. To continue developing your own practice, it's incredibly useful to politely investigate their reasoning behind their recommendations. This will also help you gain a sense of people's different areas of expertise within their scope of practice. As you work more with those within your environment, you're likely to develop preferences for whom you seek advice from based on the specific situation at hand.

When to Ask

The majority of your questions will be quick and inconvenience others minimally. You're hopefully part of a community that is friendly (as most pediatricians are!) and do not feel much stress at the idea of asking for help. If debating whether to ask, the most appropriate times to ask are when the question is of high importance, is time-sensitive, or has not been solved by a reasonable amount of self-investigation.

Topically, your concerns are most likely to be categorized as clinical or administrative. Since we all care greatly for our patients, there should be little hesitation to ask for help in clinical scenarios. Everyone has different training and experience and, as attendings, we are all still learning and should expect to have questions. When it comes to "other" issues, it is often helpful to utilize your resources. A coordinator, practice manager, director, or nurse leader may be your best resource and are hired to help; they may have a faster and more knowledgeable response, and asking others can help avoid adding to the load of your clinical colleagues.

Regardless of the topic, the question of when to ask for help is a personal one. Try to select an environment that fits your needs, know your resources, and reassure yourself that we all ask for help at one time or another. You will likely find that the answer to "when to ask for help" is "whenever you need."

Impostor Syndrome

33

Krupa Playforth

Introduction

It is not unusual for medical students, residents, and even attending physicians to believe secretly that they have somehow duped the system and that they do not truly have the qualifications, skills, or knowledge to deserve their successes. They do not feel like a "real" doctor. Impostor phenomenon or impostor syndrome is the term used to describe these feelings [1].

K. Playforth (✉)
The Pediatrician Mom, Mclean, VA, USA
https://www.thepediatricianmom.com

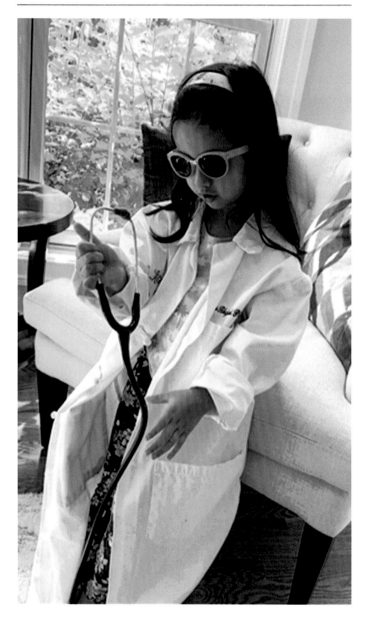

Why Impostor Syndrome Matters

First defined by psychologists Pauline Rose Clance and Suzanne Imes in the 1970s [1], Impostor syndrome (IS) occurs across many industries. Health care, in particular, commonly attracts individuals who are driven, detail-oriented, and high-achieving; therefore, it stands to reason that medical students, residents, and attendings are susceptible to IS.

Despite evidence to the contrary, individuals with IS remain unable to internalize their own accomplishments. Chronic self-doubt of this type not only affects job satisfaction but also can lead to anxiety or depression, which can be debilitating and isolating. IS is associated with burnout, difficulty empathizing with and connecting to patients, and potentially worse patient outcomes. In part, IS occurs because of the medical community's unwillingness to discuss this phenomenon; looking around at your peers and seeing them as exceptionally smart, confident, and qualified while considering yourself as a fraud is isolating. While you may believe no one else is experiencing the same degree of self-doubt, a review of the literature (and interviews with other medical professionals) reveals this to be abjectly untrue.

In 2016, a pilot study evaluating Impostor syndrome among American medical students was published in the International Journal of Medical Education [2]. In this study, female students were significantly more likely to report characteristics of IS; however, other studies have determined that males and females are both impacted by this phenomenon. The researchers found that students with IS experienced more cynicism and scored higher across the domains of emotional exhaustion and depersonalization, traits which have been strongly associated with burnout in the literature.

IS also impacts patient care and cost. Self-doubt can lead to over-referrals to specialists, over-testing, and over-prescribing. Additionally, by causing doctors to perseverate about mistakes and poor patient outcomes, IS can interfere with your ability to focus on your work, to enjoy your new job, to relax, or even to apply for new opportunities.

So, how do you combat Impostor syndrome?

The Five "R"s

5 "R"s for Overcoming Impostor Syndrome

Remember the facts

Reframe things

Reasonable Expectations

Reach out for help

Realize your worth

Created by Krupa Playforth, MD

© ThePediatricianMom

1. Remember the Facts

Think about your situation objectively. The facts remain the facts. You have trained hard, passed the exams, and graduated from residency. You *are* qualified. Don't undermine your own expertise. Don't devalue yourself. Every time you experience a negative thought about your own abilities, consider whether that thought is factually accurate.

2. Reasonable Expectations Are Key

As physicians, we are used to setting a high bar for ourselves (and those around us). It is easy to expect perfection in terms of patient care, but this is not possible. No one knows it all. Everyone started somewhere. Needing to remind yourself of how to manage a medical problem does not imply that you are a fraud. The ability to know when to look something up (and accepting when you don't know the answer) is itself a strength and a mark of qualification.

3. Reframe Your Thinking

Cognitive reframing in cognitive behavior therapy is an approach that teaches the ability to interpret negative events more constructively. For example: not knowing the answer to a clinical problem. An effective way to reframe this could be that it provides the opportunity to continue to improve your knowledge base. Another example of a negative event is making a medical error that leads to a poor patient outcome. A way to reframe this might be that learning from your error helps make you a better clinician. Finding ways to reframe facts cognitively takes time and practice but is worth learning because this skill is applicable across all facets of life.

4. Reach Out for Help

IS is ubiquitous. Developing close relationships with mentors and friends and being willing to discuss your experiences and feelings is an important way to prevent isolation. Working with a therapist well-versed in cognitive behavioral therapy can also be helpful. In turn, mentor others. Sometimes teaching or helping others with these challenges is a good way to remind yourself of how far you have come.

5. Realize Your Worth

Even if you do not feel confident and still don't think you deserve your successes, fake it till you make it. Accept the responsibility and the accolades. Do not avoid opportunities. Apply to that new job, ask for that raise, and take leaps even when you do not think you are qualified. You may be surprised at the outcome.

Summary

Physicians are notorious for feeling like they have succeeded because of luck and not because of hardwork, perseverance, and talent. You did not just get handed a stethoscope, a medical degree, and a residency graduation certificate. You are exceptional and qualified for these honors!

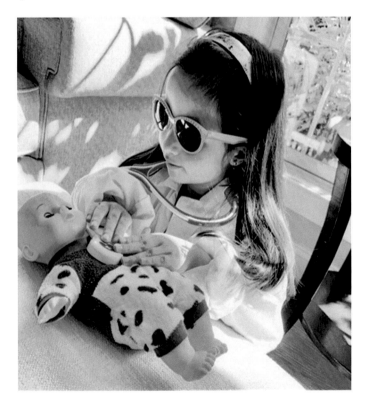

Recognizing impostor syndrome and taking measures to mitigate it helps enhance your career and prevents burnout over the long term. It also allows you to fulfill your potential.

References

1. Clance PR, Imes SA. The imposter phenomenon in high achieving women: dynamics and therapeutic intervention. Psychother Theory Res Pract. 1978;15(3):241–7.
2. Villwock JA, Sobin LB, Koester LA, Harris TM. Impostor syndrome and burnout among American medical students: a pilot study. Int J Med Educ. 2016;7:364–9. https://doi.org/10.5116/ijme.5801.eac4.

Supervising Residents

34

Alla Kushnir

Introduction

While not every attending position involves interaction with residents, it may be the best part of academic medicine. It can also be the most challenging and frustrating component of academic medicine. For many, educating residents is the most rewarding aspect of the job. By providing residents with education, you are constantly pushed to learn more yourself, to re-evaluate how to present the information that you think you already know, and to always be on top of the new research and guidelines. One of the most challenging aspects of supervising residents is the fine line between independence and monitoring, allowing for mistakes while preventing patients from suffering harm.

There are volumes written on the topic of resident education, both procedural and didactic [1, 2], so I will not be able to enlighten you fully in the next few pages, but I will try to cover a few basics.

Most residents are young adults who are very smart and have been in school for over 20 years by this point. Each person has

A. Kushnir (✉)
Department of Pediatrics, Cooper Children's Regional Hospital, Camden, NJ, USA

P. M. Garrett, K. Yoon-Flannery (eds.), *A Pediatrician's Path*,
https://doi.org/10.1007/978-3-030-75370-2_34

227

their own learning style, and some may try to have you adjust to their style. I think one of the most important lessons that residents must learn is that they are no longer in school and they are now truly adult learners. This means adjusting to the teaching style of those around you and learning more on your own rather than waiting to be taught. Most literature shows that too much didactic education does not work [3–5], just like too much "pimping" is not helpful [6, 7]. But providing basic information that is expected for the boards in a didactic fashion is usually the easiest and most established way to teach. It is also crucial to instill in residents the habit of "looking stuff up."

Most attendings have become used to jumping on the computer and checking side effects of that new medication, or the contraindications for that treatment, or even looking on YouTube for a refresher on how to perform a procedure. We often forget that for the incoming residents, this is not typically part of their standard training. They still need to be taught to learn but also that a textbook is not the only resource for learning.

Supervising a junior resident, especially in their first year, is very different from supervising someone who is going to be an attending in 6 months. The goals and needs of the residents in those stages are very different, and it is up to the supervising attending (or fellow) to adjust accordingly. Initially, the resident is a "super medical student," who is now in charge of patients but still very unsure. At this stage, it is crucial to make sure they understand the "what." The first year resident needs to learn how to do things, whether it is a basic procedure, placing orders, or writing notes. First year is about learning efficiency, and it is very important to focus the education on helping the intern become more efficient while learning the basics of pediatrics.

In the second year of residency, the focus needs to shift from teaching efficiency and the "how to," to learning the "why" behind the how. By this point, the resident hopefully has learned to recognize a sick patient and is efficient at doing paperwork and basic orders. Now is a good time to truly focus on the why and to start broadening differential diagnosis. As the supervisor, it is important to stress the need for the resident to ask questions and to "think outside the box." Suggest that the resident in their second year start looking at that second and third tier questions, not just how to do it, but why and what to do if this doesn't work.

In the last year of residency, the focus usually shifts to learning how to run the team, how to prepare for a specific practice that the resident may be joining or a fellowship. Therefore, the focus for the supervising attending/fellow also shifts. It is really important for the senior resident to have more independence and to try to run the team and make as many decisions on their own as possible. They need to "spread their wings" while still having the safety net of being a resident. The attending is there as a backup – someone to run things by and to validate their thinking and decisions. This is the hardest stage for many attendings, since it is often difficult to stand back and allow the residents to make their own decisions, especially when they may be different from yours. But as long as these decisions are safe for the patient, it is important to allow the resident to develop their own style.

Regardless of your role in resident education or your teaching style, always remember that you were a resident once.

References

1. Institute of Medicine (US) Committee on Optimizing Graduate Medical Trainee (Resident) Hours and Work Schedule to Improve Patient Safety; Ulmer C, Miller Wolman D, Johns MME, editors. Resident Duty Hours: Enhancing Sleep, Supervision, and Safety. Washington, DC: National Academies Press (US); 2009. 4, Improving the Resident Learning Environment. Available from: https://www.ncbi.nlm.nih.gov/books/NBK214936//.
2. Vilppu H, Murtonen M, Österholm E, Mikkilä-Erdmann M. How can the training of medical residents be improved? Three suggestions. MedEdPublish. 2019;8(1):17. https://doi.org/10.15694/mep.2019.000017.1.
3. Datta R, Datta K, Venkatesh MD. Evaluation of interactive teaching for undergraduate medical students using a classroom interactive response system in India. Med J Armed Forces India. 2015;71(3):239–45.
4. Shreeve MW. Beyond the didactic classroom: educational models to encourage active student involvement in learning. J Chiropr Educ. 2008;22(1):23–8. https://doi.org/10.7899/1042-5055-22.1.23.

5. Foster C. Learning for understanding: engaging and interactive knowledge visualization. Durham: Technology Enhanced Learning Research Group, Durham University; 2008.
6. https://www.beckershospitalreview.com/hospital-physician-relationships/medical-student-pimping-valuable-or-humiliating.html.
7. https://bulletin.facs.org/2016/08/pimping-time-honored-educational-tradition-or-relic-of-the-past/.

Balancing Resident Autonomy and Patient Safety

Angela Michaels

Introduction

Regardless of what environment you've entered, you will need to find a balance among your team members' independence, your level of involvement in each of their activities, and your patients' care. The general idea of suddenly being "an attending" can be daunting enough, but the factors and nuances that go into how your team works are almost limitless. Remember that all health-care providers prioritize patient care; if there are discrepancies in what you and your team believe is a good balance between autonomy and safety, then you can always re-center the conversation around that principle. While this section addresses residents, the concepts can apply to almost any person on the care team.

A. Michaels (✉)
Department of Pediatrics, Division of Neonatal-Perinatal Medicine, Wake Forest Baptist Health, Winston-Salem, NC, USA

© The Author(s), under exclusive license to Springer Nature Switzerland AG 2021
P. M. Garrett, K. Yoon-Flannery (eds.), *A Pediatrician's Path*,
https://doi.org/10.1007/978-3-030-75370-2_35

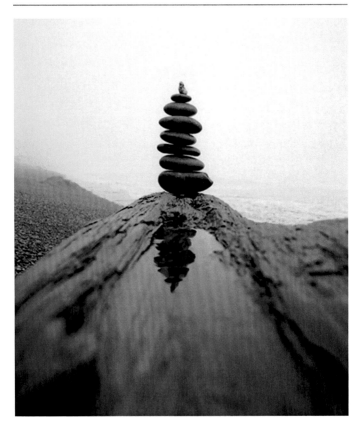

Where to Start

As you trained, you hopefully noted both positive and negative examples of supervising providers. Reflect back on not only how you felt as their trainee but how your colleagues reacted to and perceived those attendings. Try and look critically at how they achieved their own balance and what the outcomes were. Ask those you admire to meet with you and give pointers, including pitfalls they encountered or believe you may be prone to.

When entering your new role, note the preexisting dynamics, especially as different institutions can have variable cultures in regards to trainees and their responsibilities. Some clinics may allow chief residents to practice without attending supervision. Certain neonatal intensive care units may expect interns to only care for late preterm infants, whereas others will ask that they not only care for extremely premature infants but even lead difficult conversations with the parents. Gaining an understanding of the cultural expectations in your practice will help set both you and the trainees up for success.

Know Yourself and Your Team

One of the biggest factors in how you participate on a team is—of course—you! Self-awareness of your own preferences will be an important place to start in understanding the autonomy your team is likely to receive. That being said, you'll encounter a wide range of personalities in your trainees and situations with your patients. All of these factors will play a part in your supervisory style, and being able to adapt your level of oversight may improve with practice. Many physicians also notice that as they gain experience, their comfort with resident independence increases— regardless of the situation.

While you have preferences in how your team operates, your trainees will provide verbal and nonverbal cues as to how comfortable they are with different responsibilities and with your leadership. Prefacing each new relationship with an open dialogue about team members' goals, in addition to attention to each person's capabilities and comfort, will increase the chances of maximizing independence while maintaining patient safety. It will be rare that you only have one interaction with a trainee. Take the chance to ask them how they'd like to continue to build their practice. Depending on your style and willingness to "customize" responsibility, your prior knowledge of their skill level can influence your future interactions.

Specific Expectations

One of the most frustrating situations for both trainee and supervisor is when both felt they didn't know what to expect. Whenever possible, setting boundaries on what you as an attending are comfortable with trainees addressing is extremely helpful. If viewed as a form of contingency planning, these discussions can serve as educational and feedback opportunities. Identifying these boundaries also serves to teach residents what is clinically concerning and helps them prepare for situations where more supervision is appropriate.

A component of expectations that is often underappreciated is whether the degree of independence given is more contingent upon trainee year or developmental level. As medicine has shifted toward competency-based education, learners have understandably expected more individualization of their responsibilities. Trainees may feel pushed beyond their comfort, or limited in their scope, depending on the situation and individual. Set expectations and if relevant, being explicit about where expectations come from (programmatic, your preferences, their developmental level). While this level of specificity is often unnecessary, it can be an important part of mutual understanding of the trainee's role. An eager resident will appreciate an explanation of why you expect notification of any child with respiratory distress; the timing of many treatments such as steroids or albuterol can significantly improve their responsiveness. Similarly, a hesitant resident may gain comfort in initiating fluid resuscitation prior to calling you when you explain that you've observed them evaluate multiple patients and have confidence in their assessment of a patient's hemodynamic status.

A note for call-type scenarios: many physicians find the hardest supervisory role to be call, where you are dependent on the resident to know when to practice independence. Setting specific expectations can serve you best in these times, as well as having an open discussion about your style as a supervisor and their competence/comfort as a "first-call" provider.

Making the Most of Low-Stakes Situations and Clinical Equipoise

Learners are cognizant of the inverse relationship between responsible autonomy and patient acuity. They are also gaining an appreciation of the variation in clinical practice among different providers and attempting to discover their own style. Scenarios that are relatively low risk are prime opportunities to safely allow trainees to build the foundations of their practice. Especially for early-career trainees, if you provide them independence in these low-stakes situations, they are more likely to understand when critical events preclude autonomy. Helping them recognize more dangerous scenarios will enhance their own situational awareness, and educating residents on how to address these events will better prepare them for increasing levels of responsibility.

All providers encounter scenarios where multiple management options are valid. Situations with clinical equipoise offer a perfect opportunity to ask a resident "what would you like to do"? At a minimum, you as a supervisor can assess their underlying medical knowledge and clinical reasoning. In the best circumstances, there is a thoughtful discussion, and the trainee feels a sense of increased patient ownership. If you develop an environment of mutual respect with your team, hopefully the trainees will feel empowered to offer assessments and plans, and the whole group can participate in the conversation.

Always Fall Back on Education

There are many scenarios where it will feel to you and/or the trainee that patient care dictates very little resident autonomy. If you know yourself and your team, you'll better identify the degree of independence each situation warrants and when a patient's status requires your direct management. In those circumstances, a suggestion to still foster trainee involvement is providing education. Walk them through the indications for and the performance of an intubation, if possible at the time and if it's emergent then do so after. Invite the resident when you have a difficult discussion with parents on an oncology referral and then talk through how you led that conversation afterward. As growing providers, residents will appreciate a thoughtful and well-articulated approach to balancing their training and your team's responsibility to its patients.

Working with Advanced Practice Providers

36

Angela Michaels

Introduction

The role of advanced practice providers (APPs) is quickly evolving nationwide, particularly in primary care. Whether they are known by an umbrella term such as APP or licensed independent provider (LIP), or by their specific qualification such as nurse practitioner (NP) or physician assistant (PA), these team members are filling an increasing need in both inpatient and outpatient settings. You will find a wide spectrum of how practices with APPs structure their workflow, and what your role as the physician will be.

Know Your Nomenclature

Nurse practitioners (NPs) are graduates of a master's (2–3 years) or doctoral program of nursing, usually after having practiced as a nurse or bedside clinician with a Bachelor of Science in Nursing (BSN) beforehand [1]. NPs specialize early in their training for a specific patient population, and you may encounter pediatric NPs

A. Michaels (✉)
Department of Pediatrics, Division of Neonatal-Perinatal Medicine,
Wake Forest Baptist Health, Winston-Salem, NC, USA

© The Author(s), under exclusive license to Springer Nature
Switzerland AG 2021
P. M. Garrett, K. Yoon-Flannery (eds.), *A Pediatrician's Path*,
https://doi.org/10.1007/978-3-030-75370-2_36

that are acute care (PNP-AC), primary care (PNP-PC), family (FNP), or neonatal (NNP). More than 75% of practicing NPs work in primary care [1].

Physician assistants (PAs) are graduates of a master's program (2–3 years) and may have a previous background in medical care but are not required to. According to the American Academy of Physician Assistants (AAPA), their educational model is based on medical school curricula [2]. PAs receive more broad medical training and may complete the clinical components in a specific area of focus or can wait to specialize until after their PA certification.

Both certifications require didactic and clinical experiences and to practice, both NPs and PAs pass a certification exam. The description of their difference in training is sometimes described as a patient population-based vs. medical model, respectively [3]. Their scopes of practice are often very similar and can be practice- and state-specified.

Understand Your Team Dynamic

There is a common theme among these sections about your first job, which is to get to know your environment. Each practice will have differences in the way they structure responsibilities and autonomy not just for APPs but for all the components of the care team. In some hospital units, a respiratory therapist may make changes to respiratory support or perform arterial puncture; in others, they may intubate. In some offices, the nurse may triage patient calls and make recommendations on at-home management; in others, an APP may take calls and send in prescriptions when needed.

As of 2019, 22 states allow NPs "full autonomy" in the realm of primary care [4]. As of 2018, 47 states require PAs to practice with physician supervision, and the scope of the PA's practice is determined by their practice site [5]. Your institution may have requirements separate from the state, and the preexisting culture within your practice may also influence the physician-APP relationship.

When entertaining job offers, it is important to know if there will be APPs on your team, and how you will work with them—especially if APPs cover a significant portion of the practice's patient load. In most cases, even if an APP is seeing patients independently, a physician needs to be on record as the supervising provider. Clarifying whether this will be the case for you, and how involved your role will be with them, is helpful to delineate so that you can assure the right fit before accepting.

Variations in practice structure involving APPs and physicians are extremely wide. In some clinics, APPs may see patients with a single "[physician] director" listed as their general supervisory resource, but said director has no actual involvement with individual patients. Even within the same institution, there may be neonatal ICU APPs that round with physicians but document and bill themselves with said physician listed as a "team member," and there may be subspecialty APPs who document but require a physician attestation to their notes and are not allowed to independently bill. APPs may require supervision for certain procedures but not others, or they may have variable levels of independent practice depending on their experience.

Understand as best as possible what the practical, legal, and cultural expectations are for those relationships at your potential job. The physician leadership may be best to ask about these nuances and appreciate that there can be a lot of political (and personal) history behind your practice's dynamics.

Early in your arrival at your new job make a point to ask about further specifics regarding the roles each provider fills in your practice. Consider asking for time specifically with the APPs to better understand their perspective and responsibilities. Similarly, ask questions about the roles the other new team members—such as social workers, therapists, dieticians, and pharmacists—play to better understand your resources and team structure.

References

1. Nurse practitioners in primary care. In: Position statements. AANP. 2020. https://www.aanp.org/advocacy/advocacy-resource/position-statements/nurse-practitioners-in-primary-care. Accessed 30 June 2020.
2. What is a PA? AAPA. 2020. https://www.aapa.org/what-is-a-pa/. Accessed 1 July 2020.
3. Nursing@USC Staff: Nurse practitioner vs. physician assistant. 2019. https://nursing.usc.edu/blog/np-vs-pa/. Accessed 26 June 2020.
4. State practice environment. AANP. 2019. https://www.aanp.org/advocacy/state/state-practice-environment. Accessed 1 July 2020.
5. Physician assistant scope of practice. American Medical Association. 2018. https://www.ama-assn.org/sites/ama-assn.org/files/corp/media-browser/public/arc-public/state-law-physician-assistant-scope-practice.pdf. Accessed 1 July 2020.

Research

37

Alla Kushnir

Introduction

Research is an important part of being a physician and an integral part of being an academic physician. Whether you have a lot of past experience or you are interested in starting for the first time, there is no wrong time to start.

Goals of conducting research in pediatrics:

1. Provide the resident or student with an understanding of key concepts in research methodology and biostatistics.
2. Develop an appreciation for academic medicine while learning the proper methods for conducting research.
3. Improve chances of success in receiving grants, academic promotions, etc.

The first step in conducting research is coming up with an idea for a study. There are many types of research projects, including basic/bench research, questionnaires, educational

A. Kushnir (✉)
Department of Pediatrics, Cooper Children's Regional Hospital, Camden, NJ, USA

241

P. M. Garrett, K. Yoon-Flannery (eds.), *A Pediatrician's Path*,
https://doi.org/10.1007/978-3-030-75370-2_37

research, reviews and case reports, quality and process improvement (QI/PI), and clinical research (retrospective or prospective).

Once you decide on the question you want to ask, select the best type of study design that will "answer" this question. I am using the word research for both quality improvement and hypothesis type studies, with the understanding that QI/PI is not truly research but may have overlapping qualities. After choosing the type of research that you will need to conduct, it is important to consider who you need as members of your team. Do you have students, residents, fellows, or nurses who are interested in participating, and are you able and willing to supervise them? Having others participate in your research can be very helpful in accomplishing the work but can also be more time consuming and require patience and teaching on your side.

Let's briefly explore each type of research, with some of the pros and cons and various considerations for each.

Basic or Bench Research

Basic research can be performed in conjunction with faculty from medical school and basic scientists from undergraduate colleges and is often collaborative between clinicians and basic researchers. The main downside of this type of research is that it can be much more time consuming and more challenging to do at the "random hours" that many practicing physicians have for research. Time is usually the biggest hurdle to participating in research for a practicing clinician. With basic research or animal research, the experiments are more likely to have very specific timelines that may be less flexible.

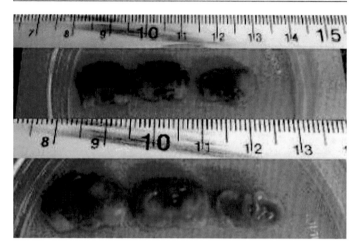

Staining slides: these are an example of basic research outcomes

Questionnaire and Qualitative Research

In order to conduct questionnaire or qualitative research, you will need an audience of subjects. Many researchers use their AAP membership or society memberships for contacts or emails of subjects to whom they send surveys. You can also conduct surveys within your staff or patient population, depending on the question you are trying to answer. This type of research can be in almost any field. If you decide to conduct surveys or send out questionnaires, make an effort to use previously validated questions whenever possible. Qualitative studies are sometimes more difficult to get accepted for publication.

Educational

Educational research may evaluate resident or medical school education practices and address multiple different aspects of educational approaches and curriculum.

Reviews or Case Study

Reviews and case studies are more focused on prior literature evaluation, with more time spent writing as compared to collecting data. This type of research is much more conducive to being done on "your own" time and is relatively quick to complete. It allows you to focus on one patient or topic in which you are interested and can be an outlet to share information on a unique case that you may have encountered.

Quality Improvement (QI/PI)

This type of study is not technically research since it is not based on a hypothesis. When performing QI, there is usually no need to go through the institutional review board (IRB) since you are not assigning patients to different arms of a study, you are using standard of care processes or interventions, and you are working on improving a small aspect of an established system. Because it is not an intervention-type research and IRB approval is not required, the project can often be initiated more quickly. However, it can take a *LONG* time to finish due to the complexity of most systems and the need to address small aspects with each PDSA (plan, do, study, act) cycle. This type of work can be presented at conferences and published. And one of its most rewarding aspects is that it allows the team working on the project to "fix" a system problem.

Clinical Research

(a) Retrospective Research – This is the most commonly performed type of clinical research, especially by students and residents. It includes data or chart review and can often be completed more quickly than other forms of clinical research. IRB approval for these projects is often expedited and does not require consents. Another positive aspect is that you can work at your own pace and conduct different retrospective studies on a variety of topics, thus allowing you to potentially find your niche.

(b) Prospective Research – This is the most stringent and most reliable type of research and includes the blinded, randomized trials. These trials take extensive time to prepare, receive IRB approval, to enroll and fully complete the study. These projects often take years, making it more difficult to involve students, residents, and fellows. Additionally, for most clinicians, a research assistant or coordinator would be needed to design and execute this type of study, due time commitment and inflexibility in scheduling patients for enrollment and follow-up.

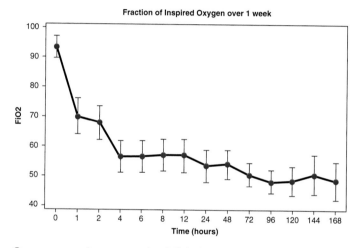

Oxygen use graph as an example of clinical research data representation

Now that you are familiar with different types of research and have decided on a topic, what are the next steps? If you haven't spoken to someone with more extensive research experience, now is a good time. They may be able to help you fine-tune your topic, question, or just assist with the available resources in your institution. If you have access to a medical librarian, he or she may be able to help with a literature search. At this stage, you should also investigate whether your study will need IRB approval and if so, what type of IRB submission this will be. Most IRBs require certification in Human Research that you can receive by completing an NIH or CITI course (https://www.citiprogram.org/Default.asp) [1]. If you plan on conducting a QI/PI project, most institutions require specific approval, and most journals will request a letter from your institution stating that the project was deemed QI/PI and did not require IRB approval. A Human Research Protection course is a good idea for anyone who is considering conducting research. It is very informative and only needs to be renewed every few years to maintain certification (Table 37.1).

Writing a solid, well thought-out and developed protocol is one of the most important initial steps. It will help with further writing of abstracts, presentations, and manuscript and will keep you on track during the study, even after a year or more. By involving a statistician in the development stage, you avoid having to learn that there was a problem with a variable or a number of patients recruited at the end of the study. Going to national and international conferences will not only allow you to exhibit your work but also to get feedback on your study from others in the

Table 37.1 Steps to successfully starting and completing research

1. Have a rough idea of a question.
2. Literature search for background (librarians can recommend databases and search strategies).
3. Refine the question.
4. Write a protocol.
5. Create your research/study team; involve those that have interests and skills that can improve or add to the project; remember to collaborate with other specialties if that will be helpful.
6. Reference managing software (EndNote, RefWorks, etc.).
7. Create a timeline (especially important when you are trying to add a project to an already busy clinical schedule).
8. Data analysis involves a statistician if you have access to one while still writing the protocol.
9. Write an abstract (use your protocol for a large portion of it) and submit to conferences.
10. Decide on the best journal for submission and write the paper.
11. Enjoy the satisfaction of being published.

field. This will assist in preparing a manuscript and may make you a better clinician and researcher.

Resources for guidelines or standardized formats for preparing a manuscript are below:

1. IMRAD (introduction, methods, results, and discussion) – Most common general structure for all scientific papers [2].
2. CARE Case Report guidelines: http://www.care-statement.org/about [3].
3. SQUIRE 2.0 Quality and Process Improvement guidelines [4]: http://squire-statement.org/index.cfm?fuseaction=Page.ViewPage&PageID=471

References

1. Collaborative Institutional Training Initiative (CITI Program), Sollaci LB, Pereira MG. The introduction, methods, results, and discussion (IMRAD) structure: a fifty-year survey. J Med Libr Assoc JMLA. 2004;92(3):364–7. https://www.citiprogram.org/Default.asp
2. Sollaci LB, Pereira MG. The introduction, methods, results, and discussion (IMRAD) structure: a fifty-year survey. J Med Libr Assoc. 2004;92(3):364–7.
3. Riley DS, Barber MS, Kienle GS, Aronson JK, et al. CARE guidelines for case reports: explanation and elaboration document. J Clin Epi. 2017;89:218–35. https://doi.org/10.1016/jclinepi.2017.04.026.
4. Ogrinc G, Davies L, Goodman D, et al. SQUIRE 2.0 (*Standards for QUality Improvement Reporting Excellence*): revised publication guidelines from a detailed consensus process. BMJ Qual Saf. 2016;25:986–92.

Staff Considerations

38

Krupa Playforth

Introduction

A team that shares your values and vision can contribute significantly to your success. Whether you are starting your own practice, or are a partner in a pre-existing practice, personnel decisions are inevitable. But how do you approach deciding when to hire new staff members, and finding the right fit for your team?

Team Setup

Bringing in a new employee is a significant decision because of the expense involved in training. Before making the decision, it is important to think seriously about how many team members you will need to run an efficient practice that provides safe and effective patient care. Most practices have, at minimum, a staff manager; staff to provide clinical and billing support; and a receptionist who can handle schedules, check-ins, and answer the phone. Depending on the size of your practice, you may be able to hire staff to fulfill more than one role to allow for greater flexibility,

K. Playforth (✉)
The Pediatrician Mom, Mclean, VA, USA
https://www.thepediatricianmom.com

© The Author(s), under exclusive license to Springer Nature Switzerland AG 2021
P. M. Garrett, K. Yoon-Flannery (eds.), *A Pediatrician's Path*,
https://doi.org/10.1007/978-3-030-75370-2_38

or choose to outsource specific roles, such as billing. Many businesses use a S.W.O.T. analysis as a first step to determine whether or not to invest in hiring a new staff member. You ideally want to hire new staff only when they will significantly impact elements of your S.W.O.T. assessment.

S.W.O.T. is an acronym that stands for "Strengths, Weaknesses, Opportunities and Threats." (See graphic). As demonstrated in Fig. 38.1, the analysis considers both factors that are intrinsic to the company (top row) and external factors that impact business success (bottom row).

Strengths

Staff Expertise
Location
Reputation
Cost

Weaknesses

Efficiency
Accessibility
Outdated technology

Unique services
Expanding patient base
Change in competition

Opportunities

Change in market
New competitors

Threats

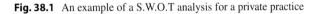

Fig. 38.1 An example of a S.W.O.T analysis for a private practice

Strengths Assets of your current practice could include staff expertise, clinic location and reputation, or providing cost-effective services.

Weaknesses Practice weaknesses could include insufficient appointments (e.g., if there are limited staff), outdated technology, or inefficiency.

Opportunities These are external factors that can be exploited to help your practice succeed. For example, offering services that your competitors do not offer, increasing your patient base in a community through outreach, or the closure of a rival practice.

Threats Although threats are external factors over which you may not have control, understanding and being aware of them within your business plan is helpful. For example, threats could include increased local competition or an unexpected pandemic that changes market demand for nonurgent appointments and services.

The goal of the S.W.O.T. exercise in this context is to analyze systematically whether a new employee would either contribute to your strengths or detract from your weaknesses. For example, hiring a staff manager with experience might decrease demand on the physician's time for administrative tasks, allowing them to focus more on clinical care, which in turn could improve revenue.

The Hiring Process

Once you have made the decision to hire a new staff member, your goal should be to make sure that you attract the right applicants: those who understand and share your values. A shared vision, along with a positive work environment, creates a cohesive atmosphere which helps maintain staff retention.

The best way to find new staff is through personal connections and networking. However, advertisements for staff can be placed with a recruiter or on multiple job sites (such as Ziprecruiter, Indeed, or Linkedin). Especially if you are looking to hire additional physicians, you may need to reach out to local residencies or advertise through the American Academy of Pediatrics (Pedjobs).

During the screening and interview process, determining the applicant's personality and passions is crucial, and far more important than their skill set. Assess their work ethic and values. If they will fit in and are motivated, specific skills can be taught. In contrast, a toxic personality in the work environment is extremely challenging for all team members, and sometimes even the patients. Once an initial pool of applicants is identified, invest time in thoughtful discussions with their references, and in thorough background checks.

A candidate who understands their own value will most likely negotiate salary and other benefits. Compensating a qualified candidate well means that they will hopefully not continue to look for a better offer. Additionally, benefits do not have to be limited to financial compensation. Especially in a clinic setting, offering flexibility in terms of hours, discounts for medical care for family members, or educational benefits such as CME can be very attractive.

After Hiring New Staff

Once you have made the decision to hire a candidate, discuss the contract with an employment attorney to ensure all paperwork is appropriately completed. Many practices also begin with a training or initiation period to ensure that new staff are able to perform skills adequately and fit well into the clinic culture. During and after this period, make a plan for frequent and formal performance reviews to help remediate issues and provide feedback. Ideally, feedback should be positive and concrete, reviewing both strengths and specific areas for improvement. These performance reviews must be documented.

When Things Do Not Work Out

Terminating an employee is unfortunate, but at times necessary. Sometimes staff that you hire turn out to not be a good fit or are unable to learn necessary skills. Written evaluations with a documented time and date, along with the employee signatures, can be helpful to indicate that you have provided opportunity for remediation and can minimize accusations of wrongful termination. This is, of course, assuming the employee has not done something egregious that requires immediate dismissal.

If, despite remediation attempts, you decide an employee needs to be terminated, your first step should be to consult with your employment attorney. Depending on the size of the practice, either you or your manager may be responsible for having the discussion with the employee. Termination should occur in private, and as professionally as possible. It may be advisable to have at least one witness during the conversation.

After a termination, other staff members may need reassurance about their own job security. Communication is an essential part of running a practice; although you do not need to provide details regarding the termination, having thoughtful discussions about how to move forward and reassign work can help the team recover and remain as cohesive as possible.

Practice Roles

The number of staff working in your practice will partly be determined by revenue, the types of services offered, and, of course, patient volume. The following is a brief discussion about the roles and responsibilities of a clinic manager; this person can tremendously influence practice success. More information on other roles and their responsibilities can be found in the resources at the end of the chapter.

Clinic Manager

Your manager will be a very visible, outward-facing, representation of your business. Ideally, you want to hire someone for this position who is passionate about your business strategy and vision for the practice and who has the leadership skills to implement that vision without your close oversight.

Clinic managers need excellent interpersonal skills. They will interact with patients, staff at all levels, and physicians and will be involved in not just the administrative elements of running your practice but also perhaps hiring or firing additional staff. An individual who is open to learning new skills and adapting to ongoing challenges (such as technological advancement or public health crises) is critical. Of course, they also need to be detail-oriented and ideally have some managerial or business experience.

Summary

As an employer, you are ultimately responsible for your clinic culture. Your expectations and manner set the tone. Patients are able to sense when employees are happy and feel supported in their jobs. Happy employees take initiative and think outside the box to help strengthen your business. And employees are happiest when they feel valued and envision themselves with a future at the company. A thoughtful approach to the hiring process can go a long way to putting together a team that works together effectively and passionately.

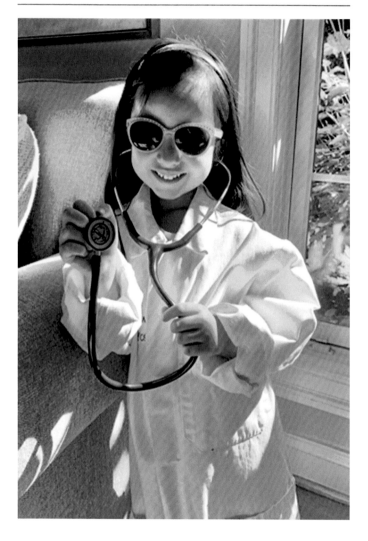

Resources

- AAP Section on Administration and Practice Management (SOAPM). https://services.aap.org/en/community/aap-sections/administration-and-practice-management/
- Medical Group Management Association (MGMA). https://www.mgma.com/
- PedJobs.org

Billing and Insurances

39

Nadia Rao Day and Kristin Struble

Introduction

Before we even get to the discussion of billing, please take note of the following recommendation. Make credentialing with insurers a priority!

The very first task you should prioritize when hired by a practice is to get credentialed with the insurance companies immediately. Your employer will likely help you navigate this tedious process, but you should make certain the job is being done efficiently and effectively. Be prepared for this to take many months. If not completed in a timely fashion, it can affect the date that you can start seeing patients.

Now on to Coding

One of the most challenging things to learn when first in practice is how to navigate medical insurers and appropriate coding. This crucial topic is not typically covered in depth during residency

N. R. Day (✉)
Pediatric Associates, PC, Phoenix, AZ, USA

K. Struble
Camelback Pediatrics, PC, Phoenix, AZ, USA

© The Author(s), under exclusive license to Springer Nature
Switzerland AG 2021
P. M. Garrett, K. Yoon-Flannery (eds.), *A Pediatrician's Path*,
https://doi.org/10.1007/978-3-030-75370-2_39

and is often learned by trial and error once in practice. That being said, if you are provided any opportunity during your residency training to obtain coding education either through your residency program or a preceptorship, take full advantage. It's a difficult and critical task to learn. You need to familiarize yourself with the codes you will be using. CPT codes, encounter codes, procedural codes, and modifier codes are just a few. What is going to make this task of learning more difficult, even for those of us who've been doing this for awhile, are the new coding changes now in effect since January 1, 2021.

So What Is a "CPT" Code?

Wikipedia says it best here:

> The Current Procedural Terminology (CPT) code set is a medical code set maintained by the American Medical Association through the CPT Editorial Panel [1]. The CPT code set (copyright protected by the AMA) describes medical, surgical, and diagnostic services and is designed to communicate uniform information about medical services and procedures among physicians, coders, patients, accreditation organizations, and payers for administrative, financial, and analytical purposes.

Simply put, insurance companies use these numbers attached to the services we provide to determine the amount of reimbursement we will be paid.

How Do You Determine the Level of CPT Code Taking into Consideration the New 2021 Coding Changes?

As of publication time of this book, the way we have been coding for the past 20 years has just changed. The new system focuses less on the components of the history and physical exam documented and will be based solely on either the time spent on the visit or the medical decision-making involved in the visit. It is imperative to familiarize yourself with this complex new system. There are many resources and recorded presentations on the subject. There are even coding calculators available.

1   Time

While previously we could code based on our time only if more than half of the visit time was spent either counseling the patient or for care coordination, we will now be able to include the total time spent on the patient on the date of the encounter. This can and should include time spent reviewing the chart, ordering and interpreting tests and lab results, writing and sending prescriptions, communicating with specialists, care coordination, and time documenting the note. Of course, this is in addition to the face-to-face time spent during the appointment. Be warned, your time pertains only to the day of service. You cannot bill for time spent the day before or after seeing the patient.

2   Medical Decision-Making or MDM

The level of medical decision-making is determined by three components:

1. The number and complexity of the problems addressed at the visit
2. The amount and complexity of the data that is reviewed and analyzed
3. The risk of complications associated with the management decisions made

Two out of three of these components must be met or exceeded for the level you are coding.

Be Cautious with EMR "Calculating" Your Encounter Code!

EMRs, can have a tendency to draw you into upcoding just by the nature of habitually clicking. In the end, if you are audited, you could face penalties unless you have the proper documentation to support your coding. This includes both time-based explanations and MDM components, as mentioned above. Keep in mind, downcoding is also considered fraud; you can face penalties for this, as well.

To Substantiate Your Coding, Consider the Following Important Concepts

Document anything and everything you discuss and examine.
   If you discuss a patient's school and friends, document that in the social history. If you discuss family history, make sure to document this. If you obtain the history from someone other than the patient, be sure to document that since having an independent historian can increase your MDM level. Document everything you examine. The more you adequately document, the less likely you are to face issues if audited. Furthermore, the patient's visit is as complete as it deserves to be. In general, aim to be as complete as possible.
   In your assessment, make certain to put in any ICD-10 codes that may apply to substantiate your claim and hopefully to prevent insurance costly denials, as they can be very time consuming for both you and your billing team.
   For instance, if a patient has gingivostomatitis, also consider adding mouth pain, aphthous ulcers, or any other symptom a patient complains of and any physical exam findings relating to the patient's chief complaint. The insurance companies will often deny certain visits based on a code, but with multiple codes, this makes a denial more difficult. Also, it is important to document any chronic conditions that you address during a visit. For instance, if a patient came in for mouth ulcers, but you discussed their asthma control and refilled maintenance medication, be sure

to document the discussion. Not only does this provide complete care, but it also helps you bill more effectively.

Other Billing Tips to Keep in Mind

You've worked very hard to become a physician and you deserve to be compensated for your skills and expertise, no differently than any other profession! Therefore, remember the following:

1   Your Time Is Valuable!

Therefore, if you spend more than 5 minutes on the phone with a family, consider charging them for a phone consultation. If you order labs on a patient and the explanation of findings will require a lengthy discussion, consider having them follow up in the office or offer a telemed appointment. Your time and knowledge are your biggest assets!

2   Bill for Everything You Do!

One of the easiest ways to improve your billing is by coding for EVERYTHING that you do and the time you spend. Examples of procedures and codes that are often forgotten include the following:

- Nursemaids elbow reduction.
- Foreign body extraction (anything from removing a bead in the nose to a splinter in a foot is billable).
- Silver nitrate application.
- Cerumen removal.
- Specimen handling fee.
- Capillary or venous blood draw fee.
- Small-volume nebulizer treatment.
- Peak flow teaching.
- After hours and weekend/holiday hours.

- Charging for a well visit and sick visit on the same day when appropriate. This will require a separate encounter note and use of a "modifier" which for this is a 25.
- Screening tests (developmental, depression, Vanderbilts).
- Lysis of penile and labial adhesions.
- Cryotherapy.
- Drainage of subungual hematomas.
- Burn care.
- Splint placement and associated supplies.
- Tympanometry.
- Incision and drainage of anything.

Take Advantage of Your Billing Team

If you have access, spend a day or two with your billers. We both still regularly ask questions of our own teams! Have your billers notify you of any denials and then coach you through how to prevent them in the future. If your encounters are being down-coded, find out why. Your billing team is a valuable asset to your success.

Conclusions

Investing the time to learn efficient and effective coding early in your career will not only save you precious time in the short and long term, but will often increase your compensation without increasing your workload. This mission will also set up essential documentation habits that will serve you and your patients well throughout your time in practice.

References

1. CPT® Process – How a code becomes a code. Why is CPT important? 1 Mar 2016. web.archive.org/web/20160511115308/www.ama-assn.org/ama/pub/physician-resources/solutions-managing-your-practice/coding-billing-insurance/cpt/cpt-process-faq/code-becomes-cpt.page.

Coding Resources

AAP Coding Newsletter.

AAP Coding Hotline- submit questions at https://coding.solutions.aap.org/ss/coding_hotline.aspx.

Coding for pediatrics 2021: A manual for pediatric documentation and payment. American Academy of Pediatrics Committee on Coding and Nomenclature, 2020.

CPT® Process – How a code becomes a code. Why is CPT important? 1 Mar 2016. web.archive.org/web/20160511115308/www.ama-assn.org/ama/pub/physician-resources/solutions-managing-your-practice/coding-billing-insurance/cpt/cpt-process-faq/code-becomes-cpt.page.

Pediatric office-based evaluation and management coding 2021 revisions. Elk Grove Village: American Academy of Pediatrics, 2020.

Pediatric Boards, Continuing Medical Education, and Maintenance of Certification

40

Alla Kushnir

Pediatrics Boards

I was board certified in the last year that the exam was a 2-day test and on paper. I had to get a hotel room to be there the night before so that I would be ready to start taking the test in the morning and then repeat this again the next day. By the time I returned the booklets and the scantrons where I had penciled in my answers, I was exhausted. However, I remember the sense of accomplishment I felt weeks later when I opened the letter indicating that I was "Board Certified" in Pediatrics. To me, board certification marked the end of a chapter but not the end of a long road, since I was in the first year of fellowship at the time and still had one more board exam to take. By the time I was taking my subspecialty boards 4 years later, all I needed to do was drive to a nearby testing center and spend a day on a computer. Logging in to the American Board of Pediatrics website after the email notification and seeing "pass" on the site was finally the end of the long road that began with

A. Kushnir (✉)
Department of Pediatrics, Cooper Children's Regional Hospital, Camden, NJ, USA

P. M. Garrett, K. Yoon-Flannery (eds.), *A Pediatrician's Path*,
https://doi.org/10.1007/978-3-030-75370-2_40

premedical studies and continued through medical school, residency, and fellowship. After almost two decades, I was finally board certified in pediatrics and my subspecialty, and that meant that I had the skills and knowledge necessary to do well by my patients. It is also a great example how much everything had changed in just a few years.

As you can imagine, these were not the only changes, and just like everything else around us, there were many changes happening in the world of board certification. At the turn of the millennium, the American Board of Medical Specialties (ABMS) introduced a very controversial Maintenance of Certification (MOC) program [1].

The American Board of Pediatrics (ABP) is a nonprofit organization that administers board exams and provides board certification to pediatricians and pediatric subspecialists [2]. The ABP has been responsible for pediatric accreditation since 1933 with the goal of promoting excellence in medical care for children and adolescents. To make sure that all pediatricians accredited by ABP meet these requirements, they examine six core competencies: interpersonal and communication skills, medical knowledge, patient care, practice-based learning and improvement, professionalism, and systems-based practice. They are not mandated but try to maintain policies that are in line with those suggested by the American Board of Medical Specialties (ABMS) [2].

Until 2012, the pediatric board exam was administered in large test centers on "scantron" or "fill-in-the-bubble" sheets and paper booklets and was considered one of the hardest board exams to pass, with failure rates as high as 25%. In 2012, the ABP switched over to a fully computerized exam given at Prometric Test Centers across the United States, with significant scoring changes that resulted in a substantial increase in the pass rates as well (approximately 86%). The computer-based, multiple choice exam contains between 332 and 336 questions. The exam is broken down into four blocks, with each lasting 1 hour and 45 minutes and a 15-minute break between each block. You are given a "lunch break" between blocks #2 and #3, with the break lasting 1 hour. Each block contains about 84 questions, which means you will have about 1 minute and 15 seconds to answer each question [3].

Continuing Medical Education Credits (CME)

One of the joys of medicine and pediatrics is that we should be able to learn at least one new thing every day. One of the ways we can do that is by participating in CME activities. Most states and hospitals require CME each year in order to maintain medical licenses. One of the benefits of CME activities is the wide variety offered. You can receive CME credits by going on the American Academy of Pediatrics site [4], ABP site [5], going to conferences, or watching webinars. You can also receive credits by using UpToDate [6] or reading journals. Whether you receive CME credits by participating in a conference or while sitting in your office, you are able to choose a topic relevant to your field and interest. On the downside, some CMEs may be expensive, and it may be difficult for a pediatrician in private practice, or actually in any position, to leave their practice for an extended period of time to attend a conference or an event.

Maintenance of Certification (MOC) or Recertification

In 2010, the ABMS and ABP specifically introduced the concept of continuous maintenance of certification, and the new MOC came about. Although, according to ABP, you are not required to maintain certification in general pediatrics once you are certified in a subspecialty, many hospitals request or require it. Also, some subspecialties require co-certification in other subspecialties. For example, in order to maintain certification in Pediatric Transplant Hepatology, you must maintain certification in Pediatric Gastroenterology [7].

To maintain your board certification in general pediatrics and any pediatric subspecialties for which you are certified, you must check off requirements in four areas [8]:

1. Professional Standing (Part 1) – You must have at least one valid, unrestricted medical license in the United States or Canada.

2. Lifelong Learning and Self-Assessment (Part 2) – This is your general, continuous knowledge, such as CME credits. You can also receive Part 2 points from certain conferences and by participating in "question of the week" by ABP. You must earn at least 40 points for these activities every 5 years, and they can be used for both general pediatric and subspecialty recertification. The same 5-year cycle will apply to all your certificates.

3. Cognitive Expertise/Exam (Part 3) – This is the "old" recertification exam. Beginning in 2019, you can either take the old-fashioned exam in a Prometric Center or participate in MOCA-Peds assessment. This new method electronically delivers 20 questions each quarter, and you have the whole quarter to answer them. Once you start the 20 questions, you have a specific time in which to complete them, approximately 5 minutes/question. Part 3 also aligns with your 5-year cycle.

4. Improving Professional Practice/Quality Improvement (Part 4) – The most controversial part and sometimes the most challenging to complete. You must participate in a quality improvement (QI) activity that is approved by the ABP to earn these 40 points. These can be small or large group, collaborative, web-based, or other types. If your practice receives designation as a patient-centered medical home (PCMH), this can also fulfill your Part 4 requirement.

There are an additional 20 points that need to be earned, for a total of 100 points each 5-year cycle and may be earned in either Part 2 or 4 activities. Once you earn the 100 points at the end of each 5-year cycle, you get to pay the fee (currently $1330 for a 5-year cycle) to begin your next cycle of MOC.

References

1. https://www.abms.org/verify-certification/information-for-credentialing-professionals/
2. https://www.abp.org/content/history-abp
3. Ashish Goyal, M.D. https://www.pediatricsboardreview.com

4. https://www.aap.org/en-us/continuing-medical-education/Pages/Continuing-Medical-Education.aspx
5. https://www.cmefinder.org/ActivitySearch
6. https://www.uptodate.com/home/earning-cme-ce-cpd-credit-uptodate
7. https://www.abp.org/content/pediatric-gastroenterology-certification
8. https://www.abp.org/sites/abp/files/pdf/moc-certified-pediatrician-handout.pdf

How to Deal with a Difficult Patient

41

Eileen M. Everly

Introduction

The physician-patient relationship is an incredibly special and close bond. It is often the most rewarding part of our jobs, the thing that sustains us and keeps us motivated. The relationships we build with our patients can span their lifetimes, bringing us much fulfillment and joy. But there will be times when we are faced with a less than rosy encounter, a troublesome request, an abusive patient. Though this may be discouraging and frustrating, there are tips and tools you can use to navigate even the toughest encounter. We must also realize that patients aren't the only ones who can complicate a visit. Good doctors are aware of their own baggage, their own unconscious biases, and their own outside of work issues. By knowing yourself well, and recognizing when you are feeling stressed or trapped, you can take steps to diffuse the situation and engage the patient in a more productive way. This chapter will explore common categories of patient and physician factors contributing to challenging encounters, as well as the best way to end a clinical relationship if it becomes necessary.

E. M. Everly (✉)
General Pediatrics, The Children's Hospital of Philadelphia, Philadelphia, PA, USA
e-mail: everly@email.chop.edu

© The Author(s), under exclusive license to Springer Nature Switzerland AG 2021
P. M. Garrett, K. Yoon-Flannery (eds.), *A Pediatrician's Path*, https://doi.org/10.1007/978-3-030-75370-2_41

Common Types of Challenging Patients

Angry/Defensive Patients often come in with a preconceived notion of what will happen, for better or worse. They may be convinced they won't be heard, sure they are in for a fight to get what they want, or feel like they have to prove their symptoms. Look at body language to see if a patient is angry. Let your office staff know you welcome their feedback about how interactions went with the patient as they were checking in or being roomed. A tip-off from the staff is a great help and keeps you from being blindsided. Try to talk to the patient about what they are seeking but don't get drawn into drama. Ask direct questions such as "What most worries you today?" or "What are you most afraid of?". Help the patient gain control of their own emotions and let them know you are on their side: "I'm here to help, and listen to you." Stay calm and empathize with the patient as much as possible, using reflecting language such as "I can see why you are upset." Follow that up with suggestions to improve their situation. Recognize your own triggers if they are present, and if you need to, step away to take a minute to regroup. If you feel physically threatened, or are worried your staff is in danger, separate yourself from the patient and ask for assistance from security or law enforcement.

Manipulative This is the patient who uses guilt, threat of lawsuit, rage, and/or foul language to make their point and try to get what they want. They may tell you they will sue you if you don't order a specific test they are demanding or accuse you of not doing your job or caring for them properly if you don't prescribe a requested drug. Again, stay calm, be very aware of your own feelings and reactions, and do not escalate the situation. Be clear about boundaries. Try to understand the patient's expectations but do not be afraid to say no to unreasonable, futile, or harmful requests.

Somatizing   This is the patient who comes in with a very long list of vague complaints to be addressed in one visit, the patient who perceives themselves "allergic" to a vast array of medications, who may present with exaggerated symptoms or complaints out of proportion to a diagnosis. They may also suffer from comorbidities such as anxiety or depression. They may be coming to you after "doctor-shopping" in the hopes that you, at last, will fix them. Be empathetic and practice active listening with this patient. Schedule longer visits with him, if possible. Be clear that you are partnering with him and offer frequent return visits so he knows you are going to stay on top of his care. Close follow-up often allows the patient to accept your management decisions more willingly and can help you to avoid unnecessary diagnosis tests and studies. And be sure to explore and treat any comorbidities.

Anxious   You may have heard this type of patient referred to as a "frequent flyer." These folks may be too scared to ask the question they really want the answer to, and so come in often and with so many other questions to distract themselves. Or they may also be coming in frequently with very reasonable questions, just needing to be reassured time and time again. As with any challenging patient, be empathetic and try to identify the real issue they are facing. Do share with them that you have noticed their frequency of visits and use that as a jumping off point to see if they are having worries about undiagnosed symptoms, if they need extra reassurance, if they are having chronic pain or are simply lonely. Letting these patients know you understand their reasons will go a long way toward securing trust, thus encouraging them to open up with their real worries. As with the somatizing patient, don't shy away from scheduling frequent follow-ups.

Common Physician Pitfalls

Doctors' own attitudes and behaviors can also be part of the problem:

Fatigued Doctors Many of us have been overworked at some point in our career. It feels like we are always being asked to do more with less, and this feeling of learned helplessness and the daily stress of being a healer can cause serious burnout. Prevention and remedies for burnout are beyond the scope of this chapter, but being aware of the possibility and seeking ways to diffuse stress in our lives is a cornerstone. Don't be afraid to say no to commitments, delegate tasks to others when possible, and take time for self-care.

Dogmatic Doctors None of us would be where we are if we didn't have a certain amount of confidence in ourselves, and a deep devotion to our own beliefs and education. But when that confidence undermines our ability to see situations from another's point of view, when it keeps us from exploring all the options, it can be a real barrier to good patient care. Identifying our own triggers yet again is so useful, ensuring we can avoid instances where our bias would impair our judgment.

Angry Doctors If you are angry about your job, your personal life, your financial situation, you will be a less effective doctor and more likely to contribute to a less than ideal patient experience, regardless of whether the patient is challenging or easygoing. As with any job, it becomes incredibly important to check yourself and leave your emotions at the door. Stay calm, be proactive instead of reactive, and take a deep breath!

Common Difficult Situations

In addition to physician and patient factors, be aware that there are some situations which can lend themselves to difficult encounters. Patients accompanied by many people, language barriers, the giving of bad news, and a chaotic office environment all can be challenges. In each of these situations, do your best to optimize the visit: if language is a barrier, use a vetted interpreter rather than a family member. If giving bad news, ensure you make good eye contact, use clear language, and establish how much the patient wants to know before proceeding. As with so many situations, good communication, with an open heart and mind, is the key.

Dismissing a Patient from Your Practice

Despite your best efforts at nurturing the doctor–patient relationship, there may come a time when you feel the need to dismiss a patient from the practice. It is vital that your office has a set procedure already established and that this procedure is followed to the letter and documented fully, in each instance of dismissal. Reasons to dismiss may include failure to pay for services; failure to comply with care including frequent no-shows; verbal or physically abusive behavior toward the provider or office staff, both actual and threatened; a disconnect in fundamental philosophies of health, wellness, and illness, for example, unwillingness to vaccinate; or clear doctor-shopping or medication-seeking behaviors.

Dismissal Policy Considerations

– Consider having a discharge warning in place in the protocols: this allows you to inform the patient of their unacceptable behavior/action and allows them a chance to change them while also letting them know that discharge will be the next step otherwise.
– Under no circumstances can you dismiss a patient for any basis protected by law, such as ethnicity, race, religion, gender, HIV status, etc.
– You must absolutely avoid patient abandonment, which is the unilateral dissolution of the therapeutic relationship without notice to the patient sufficient enough to allow them to procure the services of another physician when still in need of medical attention/care; this can be considered medical malpractice.

- "Reasonable notice" is the key: if it is not otherwise stated in the payor contract, most sources consider 30 days reasonable, with the consideration of 45–60 days if you are in a specialty or location where it is difficult to find equivalent care
- Check with payors, managed care contracts, and your institution (if you have one) regarding their specifications around termination of the therapeutic relationship.
- It's a good idea to have your legal team or risk management team review your policy once established.

Dismissal Process

- Dismissal letter: A standard termination letter in writing, on practice letterhead, containing four elements: the notification of the dismissal, the effective date (usually 30 days from notification, see above), the reason for the dismissal, and the process whereby the patient can have their medical records sent to a new provider once the office receives this request in writing.
- List of alternative providers: There are pros and cons to this – some sources suggest including a list while others caution against referring dismissed patients to colleagues; legally it is not required.
- Communication with the entire office staff: Make sure the staff is aware of the patient's dismissal date, to avoid accidentally reestablishing care.
- Provision of care until the dismissal date: Make sure to be clear that your office will still care for the patient in the timeframe from the notification of dismissal until the actual dismissal takes effect; without this, you could be held liable for patient abandonment.
- **Document, Document, Document**: A copy of the letter should be enclosed in the patient's chart, and their response, if in writing, should be included as well; also include a copy of the written consent from the patient to transfer records to the next

treating physician, when it is received; some sources suggest certified mail, while others support the use of regular mail; if you choose certified, keep a copy of the certification in the chart as well.

Bibliography

Adams JD, Rodney K, Robers LW. Discharging problem patients the right way. 4 Mar 2016.

Himmel W, Champagne J, Shook R. Effective patient communication – managing difficult patients. Emergency Medicine Cases. https://emergency-medicinecases.com/episode-51-effective-patient-communication-managing-difficult-patients/. Accessed Aug 2020.

Hull SK, Broquet K. How to manage difficult patient encounters. Fam Pract Manag. 2007;14(6):30–4.

Saleh N. The patient from hell: 4 types of difficult patients and how to manage them. MDLinx, 15 Nov 2018.

Tomey S. Removing a patient from your practice: a physician's legal and ethical responsibilities. Medical Economics, 16 Mar 2015.

Part V

Long-Term Goals and Planning

Keeping Up to Date Is More Than *UpToDate*

42

Erin Teresa Kelly

Congratulations, you are currently on the cutting edge of medical science! Really, right after completing residency or fellowship, and studying for boards, you will have the most current journal articles at the front of your brain and the more esoteric diagnoses at your fingertips too. The problem, of course, is that what was standard of care or even cutting edge when you started can quickly become obsolete. This is where all those lifelong learning skills you have developed are put to work. It can seem daunting. However, you are well prepared to do this from your lifetime of study, and it is natural to do so because of the exciting, ever-evolving ways to help and take care of your patients. Continuing education is about figuring out how to integrate learning with your daily practice and life.

Just like board studying, there is no "one size fits all" way to stay current. There are really two aspects of keeping up to date on the medical literature: learning what you need to know to keep taking good care of your patients and logging appropriate CME credit to meet your state or other professional requirements for recertification. There are numerous ways to fulfill both of these goals at same the time, making them feel less burdensome.

In determining how to remain current in pediatrics, key questions to keep in mind are: (1) what is your learning style, (2) what

E. T. Kelly (✉)
Ambulatory Health Services, Philadelphia Department of Public Health, Philadelphia, PA, USA

© The Author(s), under exclusive license to Springer Nature Switzerland AG 2021
P. M. Garrett, K. Yoon-Flannery (eds.), *A Pediatrician's Path*, https://doi.org/10.1007/978-3-030-75370-2_42

integrates best into your life, and (3) how can you get credit for what you are already doing?

What Is Your Learning Style?

If you do best reading articles, then use a journal that lets you get CME credit for answering questions on the articles you read. If you are referencing an article in guiding your clinical care, check and see if there are CME questions you can complete with it. Making reading as convenient as possible is key. Download articles to your phone so you can read when you have a free minute between things, or print an old-fashioned paper copy if electronic reading does not work well for you. Set a goal to read once a week, so even if you miss a week here and there, you will have read more than 30 new articles in a year about areas that interest you and impact your clinical practice. Other resources which you may already reference in the midst of patient care have streamlined the ability to claim CME credit for the lifelong learning you are doing in consulting additional resources to fill knowledge gaps and enhance your clinical care (*UpToDate* is one example).

If you learn best from questions, there are numerous question banks for pediatric study and board review. Look for options with "learning mode" where you get immediate feedback and detailed explanations of correct and incorrect answers, so it is helping you gain and retain knowledge. AAP PREP is an example of this, which is also eligible for CME credit. Use your phone to do a few when you get into the office in the morning, while waiting for a staff meeting to start, or during other downtime. Just like any habit, having it consistently incorporated into your day makes it easier to keep up.

If you are an auditory learner, there are a wealth of pediatric podcasts to which you can listen. You can integrate these into your commute, workout, while doing the dishes, or wherever it fits into your life. It is an ideal way to stay current. Grand rounds from children's hospitals around the country are often broadcast live or archived, and there are a variety of webinars on pediatric topics, so you may be able to tune in during lunch. Most of these are free and often CME eligible.

The best thing to use to keep current is whatever you are going to actually use. Therefore, focus on a format that is engaging for you and the ability to make it fit into your routine. It does not help you if it is an amazing resource but you never get to it or if it just feels like one more thing on your to-do list. Picking areas that are relevant to your clinic practice, and thus making your daily practice easier, is ideal because it will be self-reinforcing.

What Integrates Best into Your Life?

All of the above resources are pretty time flexible and work well if you are trying to learn in short bursts of time throughout the week or month. They can also be used for more intensive periods to do a block or binge of continuing education if your work or family schedule makes that more realistic. However, retention can be lower if you are trying to absorb a large amount of new information in a short time.

The other aspect to consider, in addition to thinking about what fits into your daily life, is how you can remain current on the medical literature while meeting your other personal and professional needs. Attending national or local medical meetings and conferences can keep your knowledge sharp and facilitate connecting with friends and colleagues. Residency classmates who may have scattered across the globe after completing training may be up for meeting at a national CME meeting.

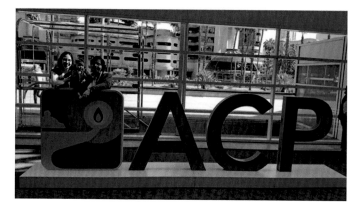

Additionally, conferences can be an opportunity to meet and network with new people. You can also get involved with a local chapter of a national organization to volunteer your skills and advance your professional resume through leadership positions. You can volunteer on a committee, or as a poster judge, or in another area of interest or passion. It also can be fun to use medical conferences as family trips; they tend to be held at family-friendly locations, and you can take some additional time to explore as a family. Babies can be easier to bring along to meetings than you would think, particularly with a conference full of pediatricians. It is hard to find a group of people more in love with and understanding of babies. All three of my kiddos as babies have joined mommy as a meeting attendee, one at only 3.5 weeks old. It works pretty well to snuggle in a carrier until they get more mobile.

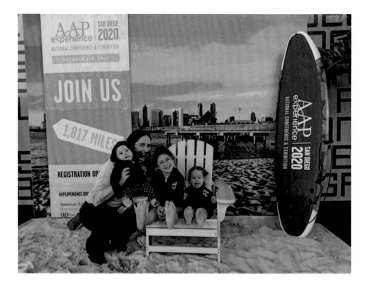

If you are not interested in travel, seek out local opportunities through professional organizations or local children's hospitals to learn and foster personal and professional connections, which can be a source of joy. Local residency programs may run a journal club as part of their residency teaching and are often eager to have additional attendees join, which can be an opportunity for bidirectional learning and fostering connections. Local American Academy of Pediatrics (AAP) chapters or subspecialty groups run events as well.

Informal Learning

Learning does not have to be formal. It can be more organic to your daily practice. There are many non-CME bearing ways to keep your practice up to date. If you are referring your patients to specialists, pay attention to which subspecialists' consult notes are helpful in terms of providing current practice recommendations. This can help you learn from their practice and reinforce and make changes in your practice. Talk with your colleagues about interesting or difficult cases. Do not underestimate your knowledge because you are a new attending. You may know recent developments, while others may have different knowledge garnered from years of clinical practice. Use each other's experiences. If you work more independently or do not have a practice setup that allows this to happen fluidly, then try to identify some mentors or colleagues from medical school/residency/fellowship who you can text or call to curbside consult or simply use as a sounding board for challenging cases.

Overall, staying current does not need to be a chore. It is about finding an enjoyable rhythm of integrating learning into your regular practice, playing to your learning style, and meeting your personal and professional goals.

Pursuing Partnership in a Private Practice

43

Nadia Rao Day

Introduction

When I was interviewing for my first job during my chief year of residency, I knew I wanted to work at a practice where I could see myself staying for the long haul. I wanted to build relationships with families and watch my patients grow. I also knew that if I found that magical work environment where I could see myself happily spending the rest of my career, I would eventually want a voice in how that practice was run.

Before I even set up interviews with practices, I really thought about my 5- and 10-year goals. *Hint*: This is a *big* interview question!! Although I admittedly didn't know much about what being a partner would entail, I knew I wanted the option available to me. In that sense, my journey towards, partnership started with the interview process.

Be Clear on Your Goal

Joining a partnership is often compared to entering a marriage. This marriage often involves several different people with many different opinions and goals. Just like it would be impossible to pick your future spouse based on a few meetings, there is no way

N. R. Day (✉)
Pediatric Associates, PC, Phoenix, AZ, USA

287

to guarantee a successful partnership based on a few interview meetings. However, the interview period is the perfect time for both parties to clearly voice their intentions. Owners should be willing to tell you whether partnership is a possibility and after how many years you would be considered for partnership. *The roadmap toward partnership should be spelled out in advance and in writing.*

You should also take some time to think about what you are looking for in a practice and in future partners. Make a list of the things that are important to you and think about that list as you are looking at practices. Finding a practice that has the same attitude and culture as your vision is one of the keys to finding a good long-term fit.

Work Hard

Congrats, you landed your dream job! Now the real work begins. This is your chance to show your practice that you are *productive and invested in the practice.*

1. *Be Productive* – It goes without saying that your future partners are looking at what contributions you can bring into the practice. This will likely involve not only building a strong patient base, but also being efficient and billing well when seeing those patients. A few tips that may increase your productivity:

   • Reach out to referring doctors to let them know that you are new to the practice and accepting new patients.
   • Don't be afraid to ask families that are happy with your care to leave an online review for you. This is one of the best ways to attract new patients!
   • If you are in a general pediatric practice, consider volunteering to give talks to expectant parents at your local hospitals or at new parent groups.
   • If your practice has in-house billing, take some time to sit down with your biller to review your billing habits and ask them to audit some of your charts.

- Consider taking a medical billing or coding course. This is something you will not regret! The AAP's coding guide is a good resource as well.
- Refer to this book's chapter entitled *Billing and Insurances* for more tips on billing and coding.

Improving your efficiency is another vital way to improve your productivity. Efficiency can be one of the hardest skills to learn when first starting in practice. Pick out your most productive partner and ask for tips on time management. Do they chart in the room? Do they review charts the night before? Do they focus on keeping their problem lists up to date to save time? Do they have each patient focus on a set number of problems during their visit and save the rest of the issues for a follow-up appointment? Since each practice is set up differently, your senior partners may be your best resource for maximizing your efficiency in the office.

2. *Be a Team Player and Invest in the Practice* – You already made it through medical school, a challenging residency, and have now landed your dream job. You KNOW how to work hard, and this is the time to show it. Be available for your patients and your fellow physicians. Be the physician that everyone wants on their team. Offer to trade calls when someone is in need. Be willing to see an extra patient when someone else is swamped. Being a team player will not only help show your investment and worth to your practice, but it will also likely increase your overall happiness in your work environment and help cultivate stronger relationships with your fellow physicians.

One of the best ways to show your investment in your practice is to look for deficiencies and try to be the one to fill that need. For example, if your practice does not yet have a social media presence, offer to start a social media page to increase your practice visibility. If you notice that your EMR is lacking in certain templates, offer to help build and share new ones. This can help improve everyone's efficiency. If you are more interested in billing and coding, offer to research more optimal coding or reimbursement options. There is no better way to show your star potential than by finding ways to improve your practice and taking the time and initiative to implement them!

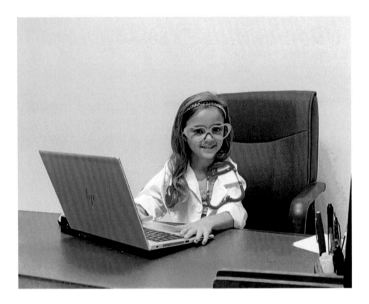

Do Your Research

There is a big reason that the partnership track usually takes a minimum of 2 years. Not only are the partners assessing if you are right for them, but you need this time to decide if the partnership is right for you. Use this time wisely and analyze the practice as a potential future owner, not just as an employee. Some big items to assess include:

- *The overall "feel" of the practice*: Do you agree with the overall culture of the practice? How do the owners promote this culture among staff members? Do you anticipate the office location(s) working for you long term? Do you have a similar practice style with the other physicians in the practice? Do you feel valued? Do the partners seem to respect each other and work together well? Are patients shared or is there a "competition" for patients? If this will one day be your practice, you want to make sure that it represents your long-term visions well.

- *The financials*: Buying into a partnership is a large financial investment. Just like other investments, you will want to investigate if this is going to be beneficial for you financially. While the partners may not be willing to let you see all of the financials until you are officially offered to join the partnership, you want to make sure that the business is profitable and well run. It is also important to understand how income distribution works for partners. Some partnerships split profits equally while others use productivity with varying methods of calculating production. Others allot extra income to partners that have extra administrative, research, or teaching duties.

- *The responsibilities*: It's important to understand what will be expected of you as a partner. Some partnerships have fixed roles based on individual abilities, some rotate to share the responsibilities, and some have a senior partner that takes on a larger percentage of responsibilities in exchange for less clinical time or more compensation. It is necessary to determine if the time commitment and obligations are truly what you want long term.

Buying In

Your time has come! You have been offered the position of a partner! Now it's time to be sure this is the best decision for you before signing on the dotted line. *Do not rush this decision!* Gather your information early and do not sign before all of your questions have been answered and details analyzed.

1. *Hire a practice management company or an attorney who specializes in working with medical offices*. While this may seem

expensive, this can save you thousands of dollars and years of headaches and regret. These hired experts should be able to help you analyze the structure of your buy-in. Be sure that your contract specifies what percentage of ownership you are buying and if it is an equal share to the current partners. Will you have full voting power immediately or only when you are fully bought in? Make sure you are clear on who has decision-making authority and that you are comfortable in your role in the decision-making process.

2. *Analyze the full financial picture.* Look at the cost of the buy-in and how it was calculated. Be sure to understand how the value of the practice was determined and that it is clearly spelled out. Will the buy-in come out of your profits over a certain time period, or will you need to take out a loan (and thus pay interest)? The practice should be willing to provide you with the last few years of profit and loss statements. Be sure to ask if there will be a partner retiring soon and how that buyout will look for you. Ask about any debts that the practice may have or any large purchases that are planned. If your practice owns the building you work in, ask if you will be buying into this as well. Be clear on how overhead and bonuses will be determined. With this information, you should be able to estimate how long it will take to start seeing a profit on your investment. *An accountant who is familiar with medical practices should be able to help you analyze this potential investment including the tax implications for you.*

3. *Prepare for separation.* One of the most important things to do while preparing to buy into a practice is to prepare for your buyout. Be sure that your contract clearly spells out your vesting in the practice and how buyouts will be determined. In addition, your contract should specify what happens during leaves of absence, disability, termination, retirement, and death. This is where having your own employment lawyer is essential.

Being a partner in a successful private practice has been one of the most rewarding experiences in my career to date. Partnership has the potential to increase your work-life satisfaction while affording you the time and resources to increase your personal life satisfaction. While it's important to determine if partnership is a smart financial decision for you, the most important part of a partnership is the people in it.

Pursuing Additional Degrees or Training

44

Shareen F. Kelly

As you finish up your residency program or are getting started in your first job, let me tweak that repetitive question about what you want to do as a grown-up. You have come a long way and made lots of decisions to get here, but there are still choices ahead that you may not have considered up to this point, including whether or not you want to pursue additional training. What type of contribution do you want to make with your practice of pediatrics? It's not the same question as what type of job do you want to have, and you might not know the answer right away; that's okay. If you're right at the beginning of a job or even a fellowship, it might take a few years to figure out what you really love about the way you are practicing. Sometimes you need to settle in a bit and get used to being out of the training mode. This question is also not necessarily tied to being a generalist or a subspecialist either. This is more about what intrigues you about the practice of pediatrics. Let's consider the following.

S. F. Kelly (✉)
Drexel University College of Medicine, Section of General Pediatrics at St. Christopher's Hospital for Children, Philadelphia, PA, USA
e-mail: sfk22@drexel.edu

© The Author(s), under exclusive license to Springer Nature Switzerland AG 2021
P. M. Garrett, K. Yoon-Flannery (eds.), *A Pediatrician's Path*,
https://doi.org/10.1007/978-3-030-75370-2_44

295

Types of Clinicians

I would venture to say that we all chose pediatrics because we found certain aspects of the health (or sickness) of children compelling. We hope to contribute to their overall wellness and that of their families. Practicing clinical medicine will be something we all share whether we are in primary care, neonatology, hospital medicine, or critical care. But our roads diverge by what we add to our clinician roles. So, I ask you again but with a different qualifier, **what type of clinician do you want to be?** When you have a sense of the answer to this question, then you will know if you should pursue added training [1]. Here are some ways to think about different types of contributions you can make in your career followed by some thoughts about different types of training that may enrich your efforts.

General pediatricians or clinicians, whether they are in private practice or an academic medical center, often find an area of interest which draws them into pursuing additional training at various times in their careers. This could happen right away or much later on. Common examples of focused training would be gaining certification as a lactation consultant so that you can enhance the breastfeeding rates in your practice and wider community, or achieving certification to place long-acting reversible contraceptives so that your practice can provide this service to your teenagers. Numerous institutions or interest groups offer these types of short courses to help bolster your knowledge and experience in your chosen areas.

Other opportunities for general academic pediatricians come by way of academic organizations offering additional training without the pursuit of a formal degree; these might be considered faculty development. One example of this would be the Academic Pediatric Association offering programs in education, research, quality, and safety to provide training and mentorship for interested individuals [2]. Most of these clinicians are faculty members at an academic center.

Clinician scientists, similarly, often find themselves in academic centers (although not always). The more typical clinician scientist is a subspecialist in a large university hospital, writing grants or doing clinical trials just as you might think. These individuals may also participate in bench research in a laboratory setting and often split their time between research, clinical duties, and teaching. Most of these individuals will have done a fellowship with or without a masters or doctoral degree.

There are some primary care pediatricians who are also interested in research and decide to pursue involvement through a network called Pediatric Research in the Office Setting (PROS, supported by AAP [3]) or in the CORNET (*CO*ntinuity *R*esearch *NET*work, supported by the APA [4]).

Clinician administrators, just as you would guess, are those who aspire to leadership and management in their practice of pediatrics. Administrative positions include everything from being the owner or medical director of a small office to being the CEO of a hospital or healthcare network. Often, the larger positions are offered as seniority is gained so this is likely not a choice in the first few years of your practice. In preparation for or conjunction with these leadership positions, oftentimes the clinician will pursue training in the business world.

Clinician advocates are pediatricians who spend at least some of their time to pursue systemic change in the larger societal arenas. They might hold public office in a school district or write health policy for a government agency, for example. In a similar way to the clinician administrators, often gaining a larger voice as an advocate takes time to develop. Additional degrees in public health, health administration, or policy are helpful.

Clinician educators are probably the group nearest to my heart. These are the folks who always want to be around learners, be they medical students, residents, fellows, or students in other health studies. Clinician educators relish the art of teaching and mentoring; they thrill to develop curricula, organize courses, and play roles in evaluation and assessment. They often like to consider how the pieces of the knowledge puzzle fit together in the larger scope of training programs. Pediatricians in these roles are most often linked to educational institutions and pursue academic advancement alongside their clinical duties. They may choose to be involved in faculty development programs (as above in APA programs or through other professional advancement communities) or in formal degree programs relating specifically to education. Residency programs and medical schools also go to great lengths to try to encourage early career clinicians to pursue these fields [5, 6].

My path ultimately involved the pursuit of a Master of Medical Education (I stopped after the first year with a certificate) through an online program. My experience as a chief resident lit the flame for me, and I found myself enjoying the responsibilities of teaching in all types of settings. I was grateful to begin the formal classes later in my career as I felt that my previous experience made the classes so much richer. Because of my preceding experiences, I was able to see immediate application of my courses into my duties at work.

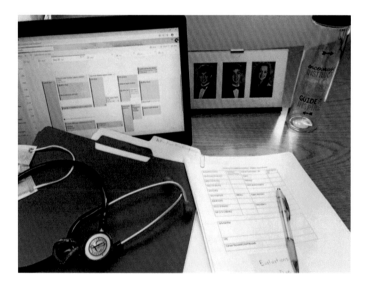

Types of Additional Degrees Commonly Pursued

Obviously, the preceding discussion plays heavily into the type of training that you will want to pursue. Full masters or doctoral degrees will be a large investment of time and resources so their undertaking must be carefully considered prior to starting. Of course, it's becoming more common to have a combined degree in hand *before* residency training [7, 8]. Opinions differ on whether the extra degree granted prior to the clinical training will have the same impact compared to the acquisition in the reverse order. We will consider timing later, but for now, the following degrees are discussed briefly.

Masters of Public Health (MPH) Usually a 1-year degree when combined with MD or when included as part of a fellowship program; the stand-alone programs are often 2 years. Areas of study are many and include (but are not limited to) epidemiology, maternal and child health, health education, biostatistics, and implementation science. An MPH is a great stepping-stone to working in the public sector or to doing research but also can be useful in most academic centers.

Masters of Medical Education (M Med Ed) This is a 1–2-year degree depending on the program. Curricula typically include training in curriculum development, research, pedagogy, the psychology of learning, and adult learning theory. A Masters of Medical Education is becoming more common for physicians who teach in the undergraduate or graduate medical education programs and paves the way for academic advancement in those settings. There are a wide variety of programs online, and my experience in a program like this was invaluable.

Masters of Business Administration (MBA) Again the length is often determined by its combination (or not) with another training program. Areas of focus include (but are not limited to) health administration, information technology, etc. There are also several other similar degrees: Masters of Health Administration, Masters of Information Systems, and many more. These programs are usually advantageous to a pediatrician who is interested in being involved with management.

Doctoral Degrees or Law Degrees These degrees are often significantly longer than a master's degree, as you might imagine. There are a few programs which offer a J.D. or PhD degree in combination with the M.D. degree. By and large graduates of MD/PhD programs end up in research, either in academia or in industry. Long-term data accrual demonstrate that most but not all of these clinician scientists remain in those fields for most of their careers [9]. Physicians with law degrees may teach or practice in either field but also often are involved in leadership or management.

Timing and Funding for Additional Training

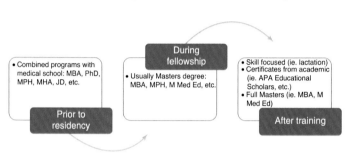

As alluded to above, a good number of these degrees are offered now in combination with medical school programs, and thus, tuition is combined. If you are leaving residency already having one of these degrees on your CV, hopefully you have gotten some good mentorship about how you can use your training in your career. The fellowship you pursue or the job you take should be a place where you can put that extra knowledge and those extra skills to work.

If you're beginning a fellowship program which has an additional degree embedded in it, you are perhaps the most fortunate because the funding is usually already covered. Your program directors will have already thought through how to integrate your additional studies into your clinical career and you should have the mentorship to guide you through the steps. Whether the training is research, education or business related, often the application can be made directly into the subspecialty fellowship.

Finally, if you're out in the workplace and discover that some extra training would help you advance in your career or benefit the way you care for your patients, it's never too late to pursue it.

Keep your eyes open for certification courses that might benefit your clinical care and make a business case to your employer to garner funding. If you are part of an academic system, look for faculty development grants that your institution may have set aside for this reason. Sometimes these monies come from the affiliated medical school and other times you may be able to get your hospital to support you by applying for funding from the medical staff or negotiating some extra support into your contract. Another option is to utilize money from your continuing medical education benefit (if you have one). Opportunities abound with online programs for anything from focused training to a full master's degree.

Make Your Mark: A Commitment to Lifelong Learning

There are so many paths to fulfillment in the practice of pediatrics, but common among them all is a commitment to continue learning through the entire journey. As our field grows and changes, we need to welcome ways to learn and improve. But, regardless of the ways we augment our clinical practice (additional degrees, courses, certifications, etc.) and the additional hats we wear (educator, scientist, advocate), a posture of humility is crucial. There will always be more to learn and know, always ways to improve; additional training in a formal way can be fruitful, and additional degrees can help us advance, but devotion to the process is as important as the achievement. Welcome to a career of growth and change, keeping pace with the wonderful children we serve!

Sources

1. https://blogs.jwatch.org/general-medicine/index.php/2020/02/im-graduating-from-residency-whats-next/.
2. https://www.academicpeds.org/which-apa-scholars-program-is-for-you/.
3. https://www.aap.org/en-us/professional-resources/Research/PROS/Pages/Pediatric-Research-in-Office-Setting.aspx.

4. https://www.academicpeds.org/groups-networks/research-networks/cornet/.
5. Rougas S, Zhang XC, Blanchard R, Michael SH, Mackuen C, Lee B, et al. Strategies for residents to explore careers in medical education. J Grad Med Educ. 2019;6:263–7.
6. Chen HC, Walmsley MA, Azzam A, Julian K, Irby DM, O'Sullian PS. The health professions education pathway: preparing students, residents, and fellows to become future educators. Teach Learn Med. 29(2):216–27.
7. https://students-residents.aamc.org/applying-medical-school/article/considering-combined-degree-md-phd-md-mba-md-mph/.
8. https://www.princetonreview.com/med-school-advice/combined-degree-programs.
9. https://www.aamc.org/system/files/reports/1/april2018md-phdprogramgraduatescurrentworkplacesresearchefforta.pdf.

Your 5- and 10-Year Plan

45

Sarah M. Taub

Introduction

When you have interviewed and landed your first job out of residency, you are not likely to be thinking about your next job. However, there are many reasons to plan for your future, as it is likely that your needs will change.

Where Do You See Yourself Living in 5 Years?

Depending on your contract, you may have signed on for a specific time period, or an open-ended contract where you have a certain amount of time to give notice prior to leaving. In either case, it is important to have a vision of your future, even if it is only an immediate one.

Once you transition from being paid as a resident to being paid as an attending, more opportunities will open for you. One of those opportunities may be to own property. Many of my fellow classmates (myself included) became homeowners, as your new earning potential increases your ability to obtain a mortgage. There may be many factors in making this decision, but home-ownership is more permanent than leasing, and while it may seem

S. M. Taub (✉)
Children's Hospital of Philadelphia, Care Network Norristown, Norristown, PA, USA

P. M. Garrett, K. Yoon-Flannery (eds.), *A Pediatrician's Path*,
https://doi.org/10.1007/978-3-030-75370-2_45

attractive to own your own home or apartment, it obviously does not allow for a lot of flexibility.

Another important factor is family: whether you are starting your own, or wanting to live closer to your family or both. Some residency programs draw a lot of people from out of the area. If you are one of these people, after graduation you must decide whether to stay in the area local to your residency training or move back home. Depending on what opportunities are available, that may drive your decision-making.

Fellowship Programs

Some people delay starting a fellowship program until after they have worked for a few years, or they decide, after entering the workforce, to return to more training. Some opportunities can allow for more flexibility, such as working in urgent care or becoming a hospitalist. These positions can also enhance your training skills from residency and give you opportunities to do more procedures.

Academic vs Private Practice

Academic practices and institutions (hospital owned) are managed very differently than private practice. There are some people who start out working for one or the other and never leave, and then there are many who have worked in both environments. Some people really want the opportunity to run their own practice, have their own say about how things are run, and perhaps have more financial opportunities than working in an academic setting. You may have your mindset on one type of setting and then realize that you want the latter. Academic centers can give you opportunities to work with residents and/or medical/nursing students, participate in studies, and be a part of a larger network of physicians. However, in working for a hospital system, physicians generally have less control about the day-to-day operations of the practice. Those decisions are generally made by a mixture of administrators and higher-level physicians.

Part Time vs Full Time

Oftentimes finances dictate whether you need to work full or part time, but also there may be life events that may influence that need. Would you need to reduce hours in the future, or want to? Looking around at the group you work with, have some physicians made changes to their hours over time?

While it is not possible to know what exactly your needs will be for years ahead, knowing that the group you work for has supported others to adjust their schedule is important. The size of the group or practice usually plays a large role in determination of physician hours. In most cases, increasing your hours is easier than decreasing.

Compensation

Depending on the area in which you practice, and the type of practice (private vs hospital based), and area of practice (urgent care vs hospitalist vs general pediatrics), there is a wide range of salaries.

Urban areas are usually more desirable, more densely populated, and have more competition for jobs. As a result, compensation tends to be less than working in a rural setting. There may be different bonus payments and offers of signing bonus payments (more typical in rural settings).

It is important to have a good understanding of how your salary will change, and what it will look like after 5 or 10 years. Will you get yearly increases, or is a bulk of your payment given as a bonus (usually based on productivity). If you are private practice, will you be considered for partnership after a certain period of time? Is this even something you aim for? Only private practices can offer partnership (ownership), as hospital systems are not owned by individual physicians. Each practice decides on the rules of entering partnership, and those rules can vary greatly. However, many have a gradual phase in or time period prior to entering into partnership, and this may impact your decision to remain in the group practice.

There are also practices which fall into medical loan forgiveness programs or National Health Service Corps (NHSC), and they have requirements for years of service. If you leave this program prior to meeting those requirements, you may become ineligible to receive those benefits.

The 10-Year Plan

Now that you have a picture or idea of what the next 5 years may look like, is this what you want for the long term? There are many factors that will play into your decision, both personal and work related. One major factor to consider is whether you are on a partnership track, or fully invested into the group practice. In general, salary does increase with years of experience after residency. However, investment or partnership track does not always allow for a lateral movement into another group practice. For instance, if you have been practicing for 5 years and have decided to switch jobs, your status as partner or being fully invested in your bonus structure may not transfer with you. Also becoming a partner in a private group may have financial obligations for you upon leaving that group. It is imperative to understand what your financial obligations are within the group practice both in the short term and the long term, as this will help guide you to make decisions if you foresee a move ahead.

In summary, I would encourage you to envision your future, both short and long term and become familiar with your contract and obligations. This will relieve stress around moving or switching jobs, and it also may help prevent any loss in future salary. Since there is no standardization or union within our field, the onus falls on us to ensure our own financial stability.

Disability Insurance 101

46

Stephanie Pearson

Introduction

I hope that many of you reading this will obtain quality disability insurance as residents; however, experience has shown me that many of you will be starting your new positions without it. Remember – better late than never!

Several events in your life can ruin you financially: natural disaster, death, liability, divorce, or disability.

Why does anyone buy insurance? Because life happens!

If anyone would have told me that I would become an insurance broker, I would have thought they were crazy. I was at the height of my career. I had recently been asked to be the chairperson of our department. I loved being an OB/GYN. And then, it all came crashing down. I got called to the labor floor to attend to a delivery. Unfortunately, my lovely patient was near complete and was unable to receive an epidural. I was kicked in the shoulder during the delivery, and she got me just in the right spot. I had a torn labrum that instead of healing became a frozen shoulder. I had surgery – it did not go as well as expected. I have significant range of motion deficits and nerve damage in my left arm. I have

S. Pearson (✉)
PearsonRavitz, LLC, Ardmore, PA, USA
e-mail: Stephanie@PearsonRavitz.com

© The Author(s), under exclusive license to Springer Nature Switzerland AG 2021
P. M. Garrett, K. Yoon-Flannery (eds.), *A Pediatrician's Path*,
https://doi.org/10.1007/978-3-030-75370-2_46

not been cleared to perform surgeries or deliveries and I was labeled a liability. I have been out of clinical medicine since Aug 3, 2013. This series of events required me to learn a lot the hard way.

We know enough to insure some valuable things in our lives – our health, our automobiles, and our homes. However, a large percentage of us tend to ignore our biggest asset – the ability to earn income to care for ourselves and our families.

Disability insurance is income protection. It is more expensive for women than it is for men. This is not as sexist as it sounds. Historically, women have left the workforce more often than men because of injury and/or illness. When you evaluate different policies, remember that they are based on who you are, where you are, what you do, and where you do it. Rates are based on several factors – age, gender, health, occupational class, riders, and benefit amounts.

Case Study

As a pediatrician working for a large university, Dr. A felt that her employer-paid disability insurance would be enough should she be unable to work. She had previously declined to obtain a separate individual policy because she did not see the benefit of having two policies. Dr. A believed that 60% of her income was covered. Then, her partner was diagnosed with leukemia and found out that their group coverage had a maximum benefit of $5000/month. Dr. A was surprised to learn that the benefit would be taxed. Suddenly, the employer-paid benefit did not meet her expectations, and the decision to forgo a second policy significantly compromised the financial security of her family if she were to become disabled. This is a common story.

Group vs Individual Coverage

Disability insurance comes in two major types: group and individual. Group disability comes in two major varieties: employer and association. I have found that most association policies (the American Academy of "fill in the blank") have "hidden" problems that go beyond the scope of this chapter. I will focus on employer benefits here. The majority are paid for by your employer and is part of your benefits package. Some are voluntary – if you want it, you pay for it. Often, I will hear that a physician feels adequately covered by their employer policy.

Let me point out some issues that we run into often: taxation, ownership, and terminology.

Group long-term disability (GLTD) vs. individual disability insurance (IDI)

	GLTD	IDI
Taxation	Taxable or tax free	Always tax free
Ownership	Employer	Self
Portability	Usually not portable	Portable
Terminology/language	Weak	Strong

If your employer pays for the policy, any money that you would receive from that policy would be considered taxable income. However, if you pay for a policy (private or employee-paid group), the benefit would come to you tax-free. There is a big difference between money that is getting taxed and money that is not getting taxed.

Most people will change jobs multiple times in their careers. If your employer pays for your benefit, it will most likely stay with your employer if you leave. A private policy, however, is 100% portable. You own it, you keep it, and it goes where you go. Coverage is not tied to your employment with a specific employer.

The biggest issue that arises has to do with the language or terminology within the policy. The group benefits, by design, need to be less expensive. Your employer needs to offer it to all employees and at an affordable rate. Unlike in medicine, insurance companies do not all speak the same language. Carriers can use the same phrases and define them differently or different phrases and define them similarly. It is confusing! The most common issues converge on the definitions of own occupation and total disability. Group plans often have hidden coverage limitations. These limitations do not need to be shared upfront. You must request a master copy of the policy to get all of the details.

The group policy might say that it is "own occupation"; however, when you read the document, it might be for 2–3 years and then switch to any gainful occupation. Or, the definition may be broad, not truly specialty-specific. Your own occupation could be held to the national economy or local labor market, not specific to one employer and one employer site. The definition for total disability might read that to be totally disabled you have to both be unable to do your job (as they define it) *and* not gainfully employed. You do not want to worry about losing part of your benefit while you are trying to figure out what is next for you – the more restrictive the language, the more limitations you have to be protected. I was told that I could be a billing clerk because I had the aptitude to learn codes.

As in Dr. A's case, the group benefit usually has a maximum benefit that is much lower than your total income. Many do not take into account bonuses or other overtime pay.

Although something is better than nothing, I do not recommend relying on group benefits as your sole protection. Individual policies can be tailored to your specific needs and situations. They have stronger language, can take into account all sources of income, and are portable.

Disability products change periodically based on claims history and world events (COVID, for instance). By the time you are reading this, some things may have changed. It is important that you speak with a reputable broker before purchasing your policy.

What Makes a Good Individual Policy

Important riders for individual disability insurance

Rider	Description
Specialty-specific riders (E.g., Own occupation, true own occupation, pure occupation, regular occupation)	Guarantees the insured will be considered totally disabled if he/she cannot perform his/her job, regardless if he/she is gainfully employed in another occupation
Increase riders (E.g., Benefit update, future increase option, guarantee of physical insurability, benefit increase rider, and future purchase option)	Ability to increase coverage without additional medical underwriting
Cost of living adjustment (COLA)	Inflationary protection – ensures that while on claim, the insured's monthly benefit will increase yearly with inflation
Catastrophic rider (CAT)	Additive coverage if the insured needs assistance with at least two activities of daily living or has significant cognitive impairment
Mental health/substance abuse coverage	Criteria for this coverage vary widely among the traditional carriers

It is all about the riders, the building blocks of the policy. Riders are the add-ons to the policies that create the ultimate package. Riders will add benefits or amend the basic language of the policy. Riders allow for individual customization.

Policy language is the most important factor in private policies. You want your definition of total disability to read that you are considered totally disabled if you cannot do your job regardless of gainful employment in another occupation. You get to decide what comes next. Currently, there are four terms used for this rider: own occupation, pure own occupation, true own occupation, and regular occupation. Some carriers make you purchase the right language; while for some, it is built-in. You want to make sure that you have a strong definition.

You want your policy to grow as your career progresses. Each carrier has money available without additional medical underwriting (if you qualify). As your income grows, if you change jobs and have a different group benefit, you can access additional coverage with proof of income; you do not need to undergo additional medical underwriting. Medical underwriting is a bit intrusive – depending on amounts requested, you might have to give some bodily fluids, you will have to answer many questions many times, the carriers can request medical records, and they will look into your pharmacy records. You only want to go through this process once. Each carrier calls the available money something different: future increase option, guarantee of future insurability, future insurability option, future purchase option, benefit update, and benefit increase.

The goal is to have a policy that will cover you under any circumstances. Keep in mind that you and the carriers have different incentives: you want great coverage, and they are looking for preexisting diagnoses so they can limit their coverage. Ideally, you want to obtain coverage at your youngest and healthiest. Dr. A had developed generalized anxiety and had two cesarean sections since starting practice, and she plans on having another child. She will have exclusions. I had to explain to Dr. A that any potential carrier would most likely not pay for disabilities related to mental health or cesarean sections (possibly not cover pregnancy at all). Had she purchased the policy as a resident, neither of these exclusions would exist.

You also want any private policy that you purchase to be automatically renewable and non-cancellable. This means that once you have gone through underwriting, have been made an offer, and pay for the said offer, the company cannot change language nor can they cancel the policy as long as your premiums are paid. For most carriers, this is a built-in feature, but for some, you must purchase as an extra rider.

There is a partial or residual benefit available in each policy. This is coverage if you have to go part time because of injury or illness, not by choice. Think things that cause fatigue: MS, other autoimmune disorders, early degenerative disease, working through chemotherapy treatments, etc. Another physician will state that you can do your job, but perhaps your hours, patient volume, or shifts are not sustainable. Each carrier has a definition as to when and how they would help you earn back some of your losses. It is important to note that there are more of these claims filed and paid yearly when compared to total claims. Dr.A's partner was hopeful that she would eventually be able to return part time.

Each carrier has a "cost of living adjustment." It is inflationary protection for when you become disabled. If you are sick or injured and the carrier is paying you, as you hit your anniversary, the benefit goes up based on the language in the policy. It should not come as a surprise that they have different definitions.

There is a "catastrophic disability rider." This is an additional benefit that you would receive if something horrible happens and you are left unable to perform two or more of your activities of daily living without assistance or you are severely cognitively impaired, you would receive a second benefit. The catastrophic benefit is not available with all carriers in all states.

The biggest difference among the carriers has to do with how they cover mental illness and substance abuse claims. It varies from a 2-year limit up to and including the life of the policy. Some carriers have a specific coverage built-in, and some will give you a choice.

As an attending, the way that the carriers will dictate how much benefit you qualify for is based on internal algorithms that look at how much money you make, what benefits you receive, and who pays for them. The carriers will tell you what you can receive. There is a small window after graduation, where you qualify for several options: the trainee package, a special "starting practice limit," or based on the algorithm above.

Just because you qualify for a certain amount does not mean that you have to purchase that much – it means that is what any carrier is willing to give you at a particular time. I do recommend keeping pace with income, as that was a mistake that I made. There is also a short window of time after graduation that you might still qualify for trainee discounts. *Please do not wait to look into this coverage.* I was that attending – I got my first policy after training. I qualified for less coverage, and it was more expensive. There are discounts available in training that are not available post-training (Note: at the time of writing, one carrier is a potential exception to this rule.).

How Much Do Policies Cost

Many factors are involved in the final cost of a policy. Carriers take into account your gender, age, where you live and work, and physician type. A good rule of thumb is that men should expect to pay 1–3% of their gross income, and women should expect to spend 2–6%. With various discounts available, that number is often lower. Currently, there are great discounts as trainees. At the time of this writing, there is one carrier that has a more substantial discount for women as attendings rather than as trainees if it is available. It is essential to communicate regularly with your agent or broker.

What Happened to Dr. A?

After exploring the options for Dr. A, she was able to obtain a quality, tailor-made policy that would protect her and her family in the event of injury or illness. While the policy had a couple of exclusions, she was relieved to know that she had a policy with strong language that would cover her for the rest of her career. The last time I spoke with her, she reiterated this message:

I only wish I had done this sooner.

Life Insurance 101

Stephanie Pearson

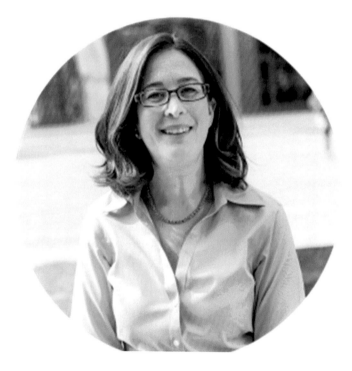

S. Pearson (✉)
PearsonRavitz, LLC, Ardmore, PA, USA
e-mail: Stephanie@PearsonRavitz.com

© The Author(s), under exclusive license to Springer Nature
Switzerland AG 2021
P. M. Garrett, K. Yoon-Flannery (eds.), *A Pediatrician's Path*,
https://doi.org/10.1007/978-3-030-75370-2_47

Introduction

When we are young and healthy, many of us believe that we do not need life insurance. We may assume that it is too expensive or too complicated. *This is a mistake.* Life insurance does not need to be complicated, and it is cheapest when you are young and healthy.

Why do we buy insurance? Because life and death happen and because you need to protect yourself and your family. We have all heard of someone passing away unexpectedly. Life insurance provides financial protection (tax free) for final expenses, living expenses for dependents, mortgage payments, educational costs, childcare costs, retirement planning, and debt protection.

Permanent vs. Term

There are two types of life insurance: permanent and term. If you are a young physician, term life insurance is most likely all you need. Permanent insurance makes sense for a small subset of younger people.

Permanent life insurance is an umbrella term that encompasses whole life, universal life, indexed universal life, and variable universal life insurance. Simply put, whole life insurance has a guaranteed premium and death benefit. Cash value builds over time that you may borrow against, withdraw, or invest. There may be opportunities for dividend payments. Universal life insurance has more flexibility in rates and benefits; you can change how much you pay and your death benefit amount. Indexed life insurance interest is tied to the financial markets. Variable life insurance combines the flexibility of universal insurance with the performance of investment accounts. Permanent life insurance is expensive, and there are penalties for canceling policies early.

Term life insurance gives a death benefit for a specified period, is the lowest cost life insurance available, but does not build cash value. Some carriers will allow you the opportunity to convert to a permanent product before the end of the term. Your financial burden is at its highest while raising children and preparing them to leave your house. It is during this time that you need the most coverage.

There is no penalty for canceling a term policy. In this chapter, I will be focusing on term life insurance. At the end of the chapter, I will discuss when I believe permanent life insurance makes sense.

Case Study

A pediatrician (Dr. B) was married with two young children. He and his wife had just received devastating news – she had breast cancer. While obtaining life insurance had always been on their to-do list, they had never actually purchased coverage. Dr. B panicked. He realized that his wife would not be eligible for coverage for quite some time, if at all. She had life insurance through her employer but that insurance was very small. Dr.B was understandably eager to obtain proper coverage but didn't know where to start.

Group vs. Individual

I often hear, "I have coverage through my employer, do I really need a separate policy?"

While most employers will offer some life insurance benefits, it is often a small policy that does not cover 100% of your needs. Group life insurance policies have varying tax consequences. And, if you leave your employer, the policy may not be portable.

An individual life insurance policy's death benefit is a tax-free benefit. It is owned by the individual and, therefore, completely portable. It is not dependent on employment status.

Dr. B was concerned that his wife would have to leave her job at some point during treatment. He found out that his employer policy was only two times his base salary. That amount would not be enough for his wife and children if he passed unexpectedly.

When Should I Get Life Insurance

If you were to die today, would those you support be able to take care of themselves? If you answered yes, you probably do not need life insurance. If however you have someone who depends on your income, you need life insurance. While that is a good basic rule, there are always exceptions, particularly when it comes to men and women.

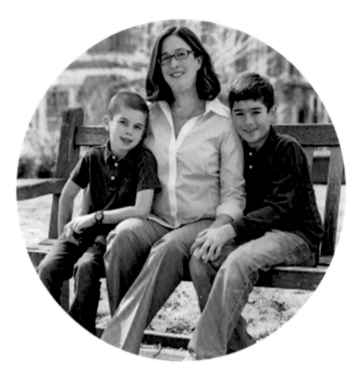

Men should obtain life insurance when they have a dependent. Women should secure life insurance before their first pregnancy. Issues in pregnancy, such as gestational diabetes and preeclampsia, greatly increase the cost of coverage. Women have told me that they did not think they could obtain coverage while pregnant. That is false. Women can obtain coverage while pregnant, and the earlier they do so, the better. Additionally, not getting routine screening, such as Pap smears and mammograms, can significantly affect the cost of life insurance for women.

How Much Do I Need and for How Long

There are several complicated calculations that take into account everything from potential inheritances to the average cost of a funeral to show apparent benefit needs. But, I like to keep things simple. For most people, I have found that 10× income or $1 M a child plus mortgages and other debt that would remain past a death generally provides a good range of coverage.

Remember, your largest financial burden is raising a family and getting your children out of the house and educated. You will need more coverage while your children are at home. Once they are out of the house, your financial burden often lessens.

When determining the length of terms you need, think about why you are purchasing the policy. Most people will talk in 10-year increments – 10-year, 20-year, 30-year products. Some, but not as many carriers will offer 5-year plans. Your goal should be to ensure that your children will be raised and educated in the way you had hoped and planned.

As you build assets, and as your children leave home, you will need less coverage. Often, people will ladder policies (multiple policies with different terms) to have the highest coverage for the appropriate amount of time at the lowest cost.

In the case of Dr. B, his children were 1 and 6. We discussed both a 20-year term and a 30-year term. In 20 years, both of his children would presumably be out of the house; however, their education may not be completed. Once the children are out of the house and the majority of childrearing has occurred, the financial burden for Dr. B will be lessened. The 30-year product would provide for his children's education and any other early adulthood help that Dr. B and his wife wanted for their children.

How Much Does It Cost/How Do I Choose a Company

Whereas disability insurance is more expensive for women, life insurance is more costly for men. Men tend to die younger, and more successfully by their own hands. Permanent life insurance can be five to ten times as expensive as term life insurance.

Rates are based on many factors: gender, age, health status, habits, occupation, family history, and more. The younger you are, the cheaper the policy. The older you become, the more morbid you become, the more expensive the insurance. You should not wait. You'll want to find a company that has a strong financial history, a good range of products, good ratings (there are many scales), and good client services.

There are available riders that can increase the cost of the policy, as well. Different riders are available for term and permanent products.

When Does Permanent Make Sense

There are situations where permanent life insurance makes good sense.

Some term policies will allow you the opportunity to convert to a permanent product at the health class you received upon purchase. This is ideal if you have had a significant health change between your original purchase and the end of the term. There are many reasons that you would like to continue with life insurance after the term product. You might have a second mortgage; you would like to help your children with graduate school; or you just want to build an estate. If something happens to your health, you are still insurable. You would, however, have to switch to a permanent product.

If your estate would be subject to estate taxes, a permanent policy could be used to offset those taxes. The IRS announced that for 2020, the estate tax and gift tax exemption is $11.58 M per individual.

Another situation where a permanent product makes sense is in the case of having a lifelong dependent, such as a child with special needs. Permanent life insurance can fund a special needs trust to provide care for your child after you are gone.

What Happened to Dr. B

We were able to secure quality convertible term policies. Dr. B and his wife can now focus on her treatment and recovery.

Managing Your Medical School Debt

48

Kristine Schmitz

Managing med school debt is more than just paying off loans.

Set a budget
"Live like a resident"
Pay loans monthly

Loan refinancing
Loan repayment programs
Public Service Loan Forgiveness

K. Schmitz (✉)
Department of Pediatrics, St. Christopher's Hospital for Children/Drexel University School of Medicine, Philadelphia, PA, USA
e-mail: kschmitz@alum.howard.edu

© The Author(s), under exclusive license to Springer Nature Switzerland AG 2021
P. M. Garrett, K. Yoon-Flannery (eds.), *A Pediatrician's Path*,
https://doi.org/10.1007/978-3-030-75370-2_48

Introduction

As you consider budgets, salary, contracts, new homes, and your new, post-residency lifestyle, medical student loans are a reality for most and knowing your options for loan management is critical. Grab a notebook and delve into your loans – understand them, the terms, and the repayment options. Just like medicine, it can be a brand-new language for many of us. Ideally, you've already learned some of this while in medical school or residency to help you with your loan payment choices during training, but if not, it's not too late.

First, let's consider some of the options for managing and paying off your loans.

Those include:

1. **Standard repayment** through your lender (e.g., Fed Loans) – You pay the standard monthly amount for 10 years and pay off your loan with interest.
2. **Income-driven repayment** – You pay a lower rate based on your income and family size.
3. **Service-based loan repayment** (e.g., National Health Service Corps) – You work in a job and service location that qualifies for repayment, receive an upfront payment toward your loans – usually *tax-free* – and then work for the designated time in that position.
4. **Employer-based loan repayment** – Your employer pays off a portion of your loan as part of your employment contract as *taxable income*.
5. **Public service loan forgiveness** – You pay 120 payments *under an income-driven repayment plan*, work for a qualifying public service organization, and the remainder of your loans are forgiven.
6. **Loan refinancing** – You refinance your loan through a lender for a lower interest rate.

Note: You may have also taken out private loans in medical school – some of these repayment options are not applicable to those loans.

Now, let's look at some of these options in more detail.

Standard repayment is typically calculated when you complete medical school, and calculated to pay off your loan in 10 years. This is the most basic, but also the most expensive loan payment option. If you have a lower-paying job (aka you're in residency or fellowship), you may qualify for income-based or income-contingent repayment options. **Income-based or income-contingent repayment** [1] options are offered through your lender and are based on your income and family size. This ultimately increases the amount you pay back long term (due to accumulated interest) but is an important consideration for public service loan forgiveness (see details later in the chapter).

Service-based loan repayment includes national, local, and governmental options. These are great options to quickly pay down your loan because it's a lump sum up front paid to your qualifying loan (reducing principal) and is *TAX FREE*. So, think about these as you consider job opportunities.

> Most service-based loan repayment programs are tax-free, so you get more bang for your buck!

- **National Health Service Corps (NHSC)** [2] loan repayment program provides up to $50,000 for 2 years of service as a *primary care provider* in a healthcare professional shortage area (with the option to extend it). Shortage areas can be remote and rural, but aren't limited to these areas – urban areas, academic outpatient clinics, and some private practices also participate with the program. It's important to know that the money paid by the NHSC has no impact on your organization's salary; it's on top of your negotiated salary. Also, there are full-time and part-time options. If you see that your organization falls under a health professional shortage area and isn't participating-ask! Maybe they can apply to be a site.

- **Local/state-based loan repayment programs** also exist and may have different requirements than the NHSC (and sometimes a larger payment, like Washington DC). But they are typically similar; these sites often mirror those that qualify for primary care shortage areas. Check out your state to see if it has a program.

- **Other governmental loan repayment programs** include the military, National Institute of Health (NIH), and Indian Health Service loan repayment programs. Military programs require you to serve active duty and are branch specific. The National Institute of Health [3] pays up to $50,000/year for researchers and may be a good option for some pediatric specialists. It applies to researchers who work at NIH or outside of NIH. The Indian Health Service [4] offers up to $44,000 for a 2-year commitment with a designated Indian Health Service site.

Employer-based loan repayment is frequently offered as a benefit to employment, and you should always ask for this when negotiating your benefits and contract. Just keep in mind that this repayment is *taxable income* so must be reported on your W2, unlike the options listed above. *Note*: The COVID-related CARES Acts allowed employers to provide loan repayment up to $5250 that is not taxable [5]. This provision has now been extended through December 2025 [6]. Keep an eye on politics to see how this progresses.

The Public Service Loan Forgiveness (PSLF) program [7] is a governmental program that "forgives" (aka wipes away) your remaining loan balance after 120 payments while working at least 30 hours/week at in a governmental or nonprofit organization. This option can be tricky, there's paperwork involved, and there is political pressure to change or eliminate it so keep a close eye on this as the years go by. That said, it can be a great option. It is most beneficial to someone with a high loan burden and who works for a lower-paying, qualifying job (such as a resident and fellow). To benefit, it's best to start income-driven repayment during residency/fellowship if your program is a nonprofit or governmental organization so that your payments count toward the 120 payments.

Refinancing your loans is a good way to reduce your interest rate and pay less overall. Many companies offer this service. Some examples include SoFi, Splash, and Credible [8] as well as many others. Be sure to get more than one quote before committing and consider your specialty and career goals. This is a great option *IF* you have no intention of doing public service loan forgiveness or some of the service-based loan repayment options listed above.

Hardship: A note about financial hardship – should you find yourself unable to pay your loans, quickly contact your lender to devise a plan. There are many options that can reduce your monthly payment, but these will increase your total loan payment in most cases so should be viewed as a short-term option.

There you have it – multiple ways to approach your medical school debt. Whether you choose to budget and just pay it back, take a job that qualifies you for loan repayment, or refinance, the most important thing is to tackle it!

References

1. US Department of Education. Income Driven Repayment Plans. https://studentaid.gov/manage-loans/repayment/plans/income-driven. Accessed 8/1/20.
2. Health Resources and Services Administration. NHSC Loan Repayment Program. https://nhsc.hrsa.gov/loan-repayment/nhsc-loan-repayment-program.html. Accessed 8/1/20.
3. National Institutes of Health Division of Loan Repayment. https://www.lrp.nih.gov. Accessed 8/1/20.
4. Indian Health Services. Loan Repayment Programs. https://www.ihs.gov/loanrepayment/. Accessed 8/1/20.
5. Publication 15-B (2020), Employer's Tax Guide to Fringe Benefits. https://www.irs.gov/publications/p15b#en_US_2020_publink1000193667. Accessed 1/15/21.
6. Rules Committee Print 116–68 Text of the House Amendment to the Senate Amendment to H.R. 133. https://rules.house.gov/sites/democrats.

rules.house.gov/files/BILLS-116HR133SA-RCP-116-68.pdf. Accessed 1/15/21.

7. US Department of Education. Income Driven Repayment Plans. Public Service Loan Forgiveness https://studentaid.gov/manage-loans/forgiveness-cancellation/public-service. Accessed 8/1/20.

8. Mehta N. General Physician Resources: Student Loan Refinancing. https://www.physiciansidegigs.com/general-physician-resources. Accessed 8/1/20.

Resources

The American Academy of Pediatrics. "Planning Your Career", including medical school debt management: https://services.aap.org/en/career-resources/planning-your-career/.

The American Medical Association. https://www.ama-assn.org/residents-students/career-planning-resource/manage-medical-student-loans.

5 Ways to Manage Federal Medical Student Loan Debt. https://www.ama-assn.org/residents-students/resident-student-finance/5-ways-manage-federal-medical-student-loan-debt.

Retirement Planning

Kamilah Halmon

Introduction

As a brand new attending, I suspect retirement and financial planning are the last thing on your mind, but ensuring a healthy financial position both during your career and during retirement should be at the forefront of the professional and personal decisions you make, starting with your first post-residency job. The bad news is that by the time most physicians can start saving for retirement, they are already behind. Your friends that immediately started working after college not only were able to vacation, eat out, and generally have a blast while you were stuck in the hospital, but they were also able to get an almost 10-year head start on saving for retirement. The good news is that by starting early and developing a comprehensive plan, you can spend the next 30 years working in a field you love while strategically planning for a worry-free retirement. A survey of over 8000 pediatricians showed that 27% of them would retire if it was affordable. My goal is that you will have the tools you need so that your retirement will not be dictated by your finances.

K. Halmon (✉)
Inova Children's Hospital, Falls Church, VA, USA
e-mail: kamilah.halmon@inova.org

P. M. Garrett, K. Yoon-Flannery (eds.), *A Pediatrician's Path*,
https://doi.org/10.1007/978-3-030-75370-2_49

Pay Yourself First

Now that you are making significantly more money than you made as a resident, it can be easy to fall into the slippery slope of lifestyle creep where your discretionary spending increases exponentially as your income grows. The easiest way to avoid lifestyle creep is to automate paying yourself first so that income is first saved or invested before discretionary spending can occur. When starting your new position, meet with HR or the office manager and automate your direct deposits so that savings are directly sent from your paycheck to a savings account or an investment account. It is impossible to spend what is not there, so by not having the money deposited into your primary banking account, you minimize the temptation to spend that money. Automating paying yourself first also reduces the likelihood that you will skip a month or two of savings which can add up to a significant amount over the course of a career.

Build an Emergency Fund

We have established that you are going to pay yourself first, but where should that money go? One of the first places that money should go for a brand-new attending is into an emergency fund. An emergency fund is a stash of money which can be used to cover unexpected expenses such as job loss, medical expenses, and car or home expenses. Traditionally, physicians' careers are stable, and unexpected job loss is rare, but 2020 has shown us that even our jobs and compensation can be impacted by unforeseen events. Therefore, funding an emergency fund with 3–12 months of living expenses should be one of the top priorities for a new attending. The amount one keeps in an emergency fund is entirely dependent on your financial circumstances. If you do not have children or a home and would not mind doing locum tenens work if an unexpected job loss occurs, a shorter emergency fund is entirely appropriate. However, if you have significant financial responsibilities, a longer emergency fund is protection against accruing surprise debt.

A good place to keep the money in an emergency fund is in a high-yield savings account (HYSA). HYSAs are primarily online banking accounts that are FDIC insured up to $250,000. They are able to offer a higher annual percentage yield (APY) than traditional brick and mortar banks because they do not have to pay for the overhead of a physical location. In 2020, the average APY for traditional savings accounts was 0.09% vs 1% for HYSAs. The APY will vary depending on many factors, primarily the Federal Reserve, so it is important to explore your options and pick the HYSA with the highest APY at the time of account opening. Bank rate offers a monthly update of the highest APYs of commercially available HYSA.

A Few Things I Did Not Learn in Medical School

We learn a lot of information over the course of our medical education, but retirement planning is not a frequently covered topic. Thousands of books have been written on investing, so this is by no means meant to be a comprehensive review. Instead, we will touch on basic concepts to help you get started on your investment journey.

1. Diversification: Diversification is a risk management strategy that involves limiting your portfolio risk by investing in a wide variety of asset classes across both domestic and foreign markets. The easiest way to diversify your portfolio at this early stage of your career is to invest in index funds. Index funds are a type of mutual fund or exchange traded fund (ETF) which track the components of a financial market such as the Standard and Poor's 500 Index. Index funds have lower costs than actively managed funds and less risks than if you were to cherry pick stocks, bonds, and other assets to buy. I recommend Vanguard's index funds which have the lowest expense ratios and consistently meet or outperform the market.

2. Asset Allocation: Thanks for agreeing not to channel your inner Warren Buffet and pick and choose individual stocks to buy. So let's chat about how to divvy up the different index

funds which should comprise your portfolio. I am a fan of the "Three Fund Portfolio" method which keeps investing simple especially when you are just getting started. The Three Fund Portfolio consists of a domestic total market index fund, an international total market index fund, and a bond total market index fund. Sticking with Vanguard index funds, below are two examples of ways one can construct a Three Fund Portfolio. I recommend starting off aggressively with the 80/20 portfolio.

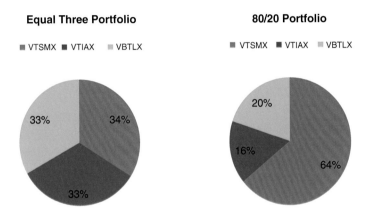

1. Time in the Market: Time invested in the stock market is more important than trying to time the market. Do not wait for the stock market to hit a low point in its natural cycle to start investing for retirement.

Retirement Tools: 401ks, IRAs, Roth IRAs, and Backdoor Roth IRAs

A 401k is an employer-sponsored, tax-advantaged retirement account. As an employee, you can contribute a percentage of your salary up to the annual limit set forth by the IRS ($19,500 in 2020). This limit does not include your employer's contributions.

401k investments come directly from your paycheck, so you will not be taxed on it until it is withdrawn in retirement. Approximately 50% of employers offer matching contributions to the employees contributions. Most will match 50 cents for every dollar the employee contributes up to a predetermined limit. Fidelity Investments, The Vanguard Group, and Schwab are a few of the financial services advisory groups that service 401ks. When onboarding at your new job, take the following steps to set up your 401k:

1. Determine which financial services group will be servicing your 401k and set up online access so that you can directly manage your account.
2. Calculate what percentage of your paycheck should be distributed to your 401k so that by the end of the year, you max out the IRS limits for the year. Maxing out to the IRS limits will help you catch up on the years during residency you were not able to save for retirement and ensure you will receive the full employer match.
3. Review the investment options in your 401k paying close attention to the expense ratios for each option and pick funds with the lowest fees, ideally less than 1%. Picking a fund with an expense ratio of 0.1% vs one with an expense ratio of 1% can mean thousands of dollars in savings over time.
4. Determine if your employer has a vesting requirement. Some plans require employees to work a certain number of years before they are fully vested and can receive the full amount the employer has contributed to the retirement plan.

Many employers will choose default investment options for you oftentimes into a target date fund that automatically rebalances the closer you get to retirement age. This can be an easy and convenient option, but the fees associated with these funds can lead you to overpay for their convenience. Take the time to explore the options in your employer's plan and choose what works best for you. Most importantly, once the money is in your 401k, *leave it there!* Withdrawal from a 401k before the age of 59 ½ will trigger a 10% tax penalty and immediate payment of income taxes.

An individualized retirement account (IRA) is a tax-advantaged retirement account that investors can use to augment the retirement accounts provided by their employers. Hundreds of financial institutions offer IRAs so it is important to shop around and find the ones with the lowest costs. There are several types of IRAs, but we will focus on the two most common types here: the traditional IRA and the Roth IRA. Both IRAs have the same contribution amount, $6000 for 2020, set by the IRS on a yearly basis. The main difference between the two IRAs is how they are taxed.

Traditional IRAs are tax-deferred retirement accounts similar to 401ks in that individuals can invest pre-tax money to a retirement account where the money grows tax deferred until withdrawal during retirement. The withdrawals are then taxed at your current income rate during retirement. Traditional IRAs can be tax deductible, but if you also contribute to an employer-sponsored retirement plan, the amount you can deduct will be dependent on your modified adjusted gross income. Although pediatrics is not one of the highly compensated specialties, most pediatricians will still make too much money to take advantage of the tax deduction.

Roth IRAs differ from traditional IRAs in that the contributions are made from after tax dollars, so all investments grow without any taxes on the gains and when you retire, you can withdraw from a Roth IRA without incurring any income tax. Most physicians will be in a higher tax bracket at retirement than early in their career, so investing in Roth IRAs is a great way to minimize your tax bill in retirement. I know you are probably wondering, "why doesn't everyone just contribute to a Roth IRA? They sound too good to be true." Well, the answer is because the IRS has income limits above which you cannot contribute to a Roth IRA. Make sure in the first year post residency, you fully fund a Roth IRA. When your income exceeds the limits to contribute to a Roth IRA, you can still fund one via an entity known as the "Backdoor Roth" during which you fund a traditional IRA and then immediately convert it to a Roth IRA. Backdoor Roth IRAs are more complicated than the intended scope of this chapter so instead of going too far in the weeds, I recommend you read more on the topic and keep it in the back of your mind as an option.

This is, by no means, an exhaustive review of all of the financial tools at your fingertips when it comes to financial planning and retirement. There are health savings accounts, taxable accounts, and SEP IRAs to name a few which can serve as other ways to prepare for retirement. I will frequently give medical students and residents the feedback to continue to read to expand their knowledge base. I hope this chapter gave you a foundation upon which you can continue to read, grow, and have both a successful professional career and a successful, stress free retirement.

Suggested Reading

Dahle JM. The white coat investor: a doctor's guide to personal finance and investing. White Coat Investor LLC; 2014.
Doroghazi R. The physician's guide to investing: a practical approach to building wealth. Humana; 2007.

Switching Jobs

50

Sarah M. Taub

Introduction

Changing jobs in healthcare is unique to other industries; however, it can be done. I will describe below some areas to consider during this process. And to give you my background, I moved from private practice to two different hospital-based practices and that also included an interstate move.

Work Out What You Want

No matter how much pleasure you find in your job, we all have tough times that make us wonder if working at another institution or practice will be better. Before you take the leap, think about what you want in your new role. Are you feeling stressed with hours or shift work and want a job that has more flexibility? Do you want an opportunity to travel, or teach? Or is it a better salary that you are looking for?

Do your research into your new job and make sure your current clinical skill level is up to par. Networking will be key in finding future positions and often is the best way to find open positions. Keep in touch with your colleagues and mentors from residency

S. M. Taub (✉)
Children's Hospital of Philadelphia, Care Network Norristown, Norristown, PA, USA

© The Author(s), under exclusive license to Springer Nature Switzerland AG 2021
P. M. Garrett, K. Yoon-Flannery (eds.), *A Pediatrician's Path*,
https://doi.org/10.1007/978-3-030-75370-2_50

and beyond, you will find them invaluable assets during your job search.

Contracts

We are bound by contracts, and usually within those contracts are restrictive covenants. A restrictive covenant describes the radial area within which you are restricted from practicing, usually within a certain time frame from leaving the practice. For instance, you may have a 5, 10, 25, or more mile radius for any number of years after you leave that position. This is important because you may be sued by your old employer, and your potential new employer may not want to take on that risk. Despite what some people may tell you, physicians can spend a lot of time and money on litigation in these cases, and it is advisable to avoid this situation if at all possible.

When looking to sign your new contract, I would encourage you to know your worth. There is a standard that many look to, the MGMA standard. This is a compiled database to help healthcare professionals assess their salaries in the marketplace. This database is extremely useful and provides salaries across disciplines and areas of the country.

Interviewing

Just as in residency, there is an interview process and submission of references for your new job. Depending on how much time has elapsed since residency, you may be able to use some people from your residency program. If it has been 5 years or more, you will likely need someone at your current practice to give you a reference. Many people do interview anonymously and use one or two colleagues who can be trusted and will support your job change. Other times, you may be leaving for a timed move, and in that case it is best to use your senior most physician (who you are sure will give you a good reference).

I found that the second (or more) time around, the interview process is not only for your future employer but also to your benefit. At this stage, you have more knowledge and experience about how practices are run, and you may also be looking for certain changes. Make sure to have a good list of questions going into the interview and compare and contrast to what you are already doing in your current practice.

What will be foremost on their mind when interviewing you is this question: *why do you want to leave*? Make sure you know the answer to this question before they ask, as this will drive their first impression. If there were personal conflicts rather than practice-related issues, this will be a red flag for future employers.

Giving Notice

Now that you have interviewed and found your new position (and maybe even signed a contract), it is time to inform your employer. This conversation is never easy, but there are ways to make it more pleasant and hopefully leave you on good terms.

First of all, give your employer the appropriate amount of notice, at least that which is stated in your contract. The time period prior to leaving is a time for your employer to reassign schedules and possibly hire another employee. In fairness to your patients, it also allows you to give families enough notice about your departure.

When discussing your reasons for leaving, never make it personal. Always keep a professional explanation, even if there were some personal riffs. I have found that the pediatric community can be small, and when bridges are burned, oftentimes the word gets out. In addition, you may need their recommendations at a future time.

Starting Anew

When practices are hiring more experienced physicians, they will have expectations that you will be able to ramp up your practice faster than if you had just left residency. However, you may be working with a new EHR system, and definitely with new staff. Make sure to take the time you need to adjust and not burn yourself out at the start.

Be upfront about any vacations that you have already planned, or medical leave. The last thing you want to do is start on the wrong foot.

Moving Out of State

If you are moving to another state, make sure that you have all of your state licensure available and ready for a reappointment. When you are applying for privileges at hospitals, it can take months to be certified. Make sure to keep all of your documentation at hand for these applications.

Future Looks Bright

Thinking about leaving your job can be stressful and scary. You may have worked there for several years, and have good friends as colleagues, and likely have a following of families. From my experience, I know that in that moment, it feels that you may be making the wrong decision. However, what made you start looking for a change in the first place? Now that I have the capability of hindsight, I can say without a doubt that making the job changes also made me a happier person and a better pediatrician. We often learn what we enjoy the most, by being exposed to what we like the least. So do not feel guilty about leaving (as we all do), because if you had wanted to stay, you likely would have.

Your Side Hustle

51

Parisa M. Garrett

Introduction

Let's face it: you didn't go into pediatrics for the money. No one does. Pediatrics is consistently ranked as one of the least lucrative fields of medicine, with average salaries less than half that of top paying specialties [1]. Of course, the rewards of pediatrics are plentiful, and compensation is still well above that of the average American [2]. However, there may come a point in your career at which you decide to explore additional sources of income. Enter your side hustle.

As physicians, our rigorous education and training are structured in a way that makes it difficult to focus on anything else. Outside interests are often pushed aside as efforts to optimize our education and medical career take center stage. When we finally emerge from the blur of medical school, residency, and fellowship, we have been so conditioned to direct our attention to the next steps in our career that it doesn't even occur to us that there may be other avenues by which to generate income.

P. M. Garrett (✉)
Philadelphia Department of Public Health, Ambulatory Health Services, Philadelphia, PA, USA
e-mail: parisa.garrett@phila.gov

© The Author(s), under exclusive license to Springer Nature Switzerland AG 2021
P. M. Garrett, K. Yoon-Flannery (eds.), *A Pediatrician's Path*,
https://doi.org/10.1007/978-3-030-75370-2_51

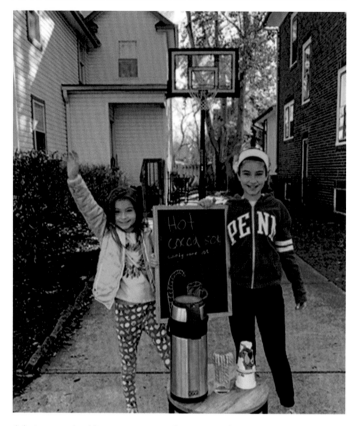

A hot cocoa stand is one way to supplement your income

Of course, taking on more responsibility or extending your hours at your day job is one method of increasing your earnings. However, other opportunities do exist for physicians, and these may offer more flexibility and a less demanding environment than the practice of traditional clinical medicine. Aside from the obvious benefits of earning extra income, there may be tax benefits as well. If you earn more than a predetermined dollar amount in a calendar year, you will likely be able to deduct certain business expenses from your tax bill. However, you may also be required to pay self-employment taxes; consultation with an accountant is suggested. A discussion of all options for additional income is beyond the scope of this chapter, but we will touch upon some of the more common side hustles for pediatricians.

Surveys/Focus Groups

Medical surveys and focus groups are easy ways to generate income during your downtime, as researchers and marketing companies are often willing to pay a premium in exchange for the opinion of a physician [3]. You may be asked to participate online, by telephone or video, or in-person, and topics may include vaccines, new devices, or medications. The time commitment may range from 5 minutes for a quick online survey to a 2-hour in-person interview. Compensation offered is variable, and you will have to decide whether an opportunity is worth your time. I have found that many companies are willing to pay general pediatricians on average $250–$350 for 1 hour, and subspecialists may earn more. Registering with a company will put you in their database, and they will contact you as opportunities become available.

Medical Writing

Medical writing encompasses a variety of different opportunities – pediatricians may consider writing a blog, writing board review questions, writing for medical publications, or writing for a pharmaceutical company about a new drug. Compensation is highly variable – for example, I have seen different board review companies offer anywhere from $12 to $75 per question. Revenue from blogging is typically dependent upon advertisers or product sales, while income generated from commissioned writing for publications and board review companies is likely to be a predetermined fee. Either way, compensation for the effort and time spent writing is unlikely to be comparable to your hourly rate as an attending. However, writing can be done at home, on your own time, and by facilitating creativity and self-expression it may provide a certain fulfillment that is difficult to achieve through clinical medicine.

Speaking

If you enjoy public speaking and have a specific expertise in a popular or relevant topic, you may consider marketing yourself for speaking engagements. A good speaker typically is both knowledgeable and passionate about their topic. Establishing yourself as a speaker may involve networking, promoting yourself on social media or job networking websites, or developing a website. As with other side hustles, the time commitment and compensation vary widely depending on the audience and forum. Some engagements may require a flight, hotel stay, and childcare at home, while others are local and require only a few hours of your time. You can set your fee based upon these factors, deciding what makes the commitment worthwhile for you. Speaking for free may even be beneficial while you are establishing yourself as a speaker, as publicity received from an event may help propel your reputation.

Chart Review

Second opinions regarding patient management are often sought by insurance companies, independent review organizations, and hospitals. The work involves reviewing patient charts and making recommendations regarding issues such as medical management, medical necessity, length of stay, and procedures. Signing up with independent review organizations allows companies to contact you based on your field of expertise. Demand varies by specialty, as does compensation, with average rates approximately 50–100% of your hourly clinical rate. More information can be found on the website for the National Association of Independent Review Organizations.

Expert Witness

Lawyers often seek expert medical advice to support their claims in court. As an expert witness, you will be asked to review a medical record and then answer questions from the lawyers involved in the case. Enrolling in one of the many databases of expert witnesses and designating your field(s) of expertise allows lawyers to contact you. Working as an expert witness is typically more lucrative than working as a pediatrician, and you are able to negotiate your fee for each case that you handle [4].

Real Estate

Not all avenues of revenue need to be related to your medical degree. Many physicians have found real estate investment to be a worthwhile endeavor with significant rewards. There are many possibilities within this category – you can own your own properties, invest in crowdfunding or group syndication, or invest in real estate investment trusts (REITs) [5]. If owning, you can explore different types of properties including apartment buildings, single family homes, or commercial properties. You can be full owner or part owner. Your property may increase in value over time, and you may be able to earn passive income by renting it. Property can be passed on to your children or used as collateral. Crowdfunding and group syndication allow for more passive involvement with smaller sums of money, without the hassle that comes with owning property outright. REITs are bought and sold like other stock through a brokerage account [6].

These are just a few of the many options available to generate additional income as a pediatrician. Other avenues for income include, but are not limited to, telemedicine, consulting, medical spas, locum tenens, app development, medical technology, product development, and stock market investing. To read about additional opportunities, or to further explore one of the ideas mentioned above, check out the sites below [7]. Good luck and happy earning!

References

1. Kane L. Medscape physician compensation report 2020. 2020. https://www.medscape.com/slideshow/2020-compensation-overview-6012684. Accessed 23 Oct 2020.
2. Measures of Central Tendency for Wage Data. Social Security Administration. 2019. https://www.ssa.gov/oact/cola/central.html. Accessed 23 Oct 2020.
3. Janoff C. 8 side hustles for doctors. Finity Group, LLC. 2019. https://thefinitygroup.com/blog/8-side-hustles-for-doctors. Accessed 30 Nov 2020.
4. Beran D. 7 physician side hustles. White Coat Investor. 2019. https://www.whitecoatinvestor.com/7-physician-side-hustles/. Accessed 17 Nov 2020.
5. Mehta N. Physician side gigs. 2019. https://www.physiciansidegigs.com/. Accessed 17 Nov 2020.
6. Voigt K. REITs: what they are and how to invest in them. Nerdwallet 2020. https://www.nerdwallet.com/article/investing/reit-investing. Accessed 18 Dec 2020.
7. SEAK Physician Resources. https://seak.com/physician-resources/. Accessed 17 Nov 2020.

Your Online Presence

52

Joannie Yeh

Mingling at the Cocktail Party

An article that is tweeted repeatedly is 11 times more likely to be cited than an article with fewer tweets [1]. Another study shows that an article shared through various social media platforms (Twitter, Facebook, or LinkedIn) boosted website visits to the article versus minimal visits with no social media shares [2]. As a healthcare professional, having a social media presence can be very powerful in helping people learn about your work and your expertise and in helping you learn about the latest research and policies related to your specialty. Here are some statistics showing who's on social media and what they are using it for [3]:

- 2.65 billion people worldwide
- 70% of Americans
- 33% of patients search online for information about treatments
- 80% of doctors, with about half of them using social media for professional purposes

J. Yeh (✉)
Sidney Kimmel Medical College, Philadelphia, PA, USA
http://www.betamomma.com/

© The Author(s), under exclusive license to Springer Nature
Switzerland AG 2021
P. M. Garrett, K. Yoon-Flannery (eds.), *A Pediatrician's Path*,
https://doi.org/10.1007/978-3-030-75370-2_52

Go to where the people are hanging out. Join the giant, world-wide cocktail party.

- *Do you hear someone saying they heard from a friend of a friend that their daughter had a reaction from the HPV vaccine?* Join the conversation to share safety data from a study or your own blog post about dispelling common myths about the HPV vaccine.
- *Was there some huge update that you want everyone to know about, like how the HPV vaccine used to be three doses and is now just as effective in two doses for certain ages?* Start a conversation about it by sharing a graphic from the CDC or your own article on HPV vaccine updates.
- *Did you do research on HPV vaccine rates in your practice?* Start a conversation to tell other doctors about it by sharing your publication link and by inviting podcast hosts and magazine writers to interview you about it.
- *Do you see people dancing?* Walk toward them and share your moves!

The reasons to engage in social media are plenty. You can share evidence-based information with other doctors or with people who are like your patients. You can learn from other doctors about their research or about highlights from conferences you can't attend in person. You can exchange stories about experiences you have had first hand and stories from patients. You can also find mentors and connect with people who may end up inviting you to be a speaker or to collaborate on a project together. Let's break down the steps on how to start to mingle and how to curate a network that can help you move your career forward.

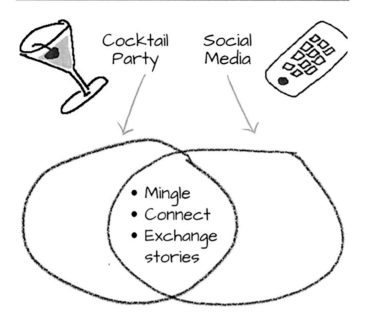

Create Your Online Footprint

Have you ever searched your name on the internet? Try it. What are the first ten results? How much of those results are content created *by you* versus a profile assembled *for you* by a health company? Here's the thing. Patients, potential collaborators, potential employers, and many others will Google you. Make it easy for people to find you. Be in control of what is written about you by creating your own footprint. Be patient, because this process takes time and your approach may evolve over time, too, but the key point is to just get started.

Pick three to five main medical topics and two to three fun topics you want to post about often. When you create profiles on platforms like LinkedIn, Doximity, your practice website, or Twitter, mention these interests. Share articles, infographics, and tips related to these areas. Mention to everyone you talk to that these are the topics that you are passionate about. If a news reporter asked your practice or communications manager who to interview about those topics, that manager should be able to reflexively respond with your name. Eventually, as you write and speak about them, search engines will also reflexively respond with your name attached to these topics.

Platforms and Purpose

So where is this cocktail party? It's actually happening in a few places all at once, but you don't have to be omnipresent. Pick one or two platforms to explore. Get accustomed to the language (e.g., hashtags), the other guests (who do you want to follow, who should you report and block?), and the flow of the space. Take time to make new friends there. Chances are they can be your friends when you are ready to try out other platforms, too. You may already have a personal TikTok or Instagram account, but I recommend starting on Twitter to start making professional connections. Once you are comfortable, you can also make profiles in your hospital system's directory, Doximity, Pinterest, TikTok, or Instagram.

Let's review how we can be an ace at the cocktail party. We will use the ACE mnemonic which stands for Advocate, Collaborate, and Educate. These activities provide a framework for how to be intentional in making connections, starting and joining converations, and finding friends and an audience on these platforms.

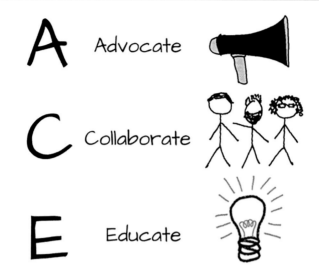

- Advocate
  - Share which congressional bills can better serve your patients.
  - Connect with key stakeholders and legislators.
  - Share stories of how patients are affected by policies.
- Collaborate
  - Meet mentors, mentees, and sponsors.
  - Find partners to work with on writing, advocacy, or research projects.
  - Get invited to conferences and hospitals to speak on your area of expertise.

- Educate
  - Share research findings and news on three to five core topics.
  - Learn from patients sharing their stories.
  - Learn from other healthcare workers anywhere in the world.

Connect and Engage

So, if social media is a cocktail party, what should you wear? Posting content is like getting dressed. You wouldn't leave home naked, right? Well then, don't start approaching people at the party before you have put on some clothes (i.e., content). People will be more likely to follow you if they are able to get a sense of your background and personality.

Take a few photos of yourself and a few photos of random things that mean something to you, such as a coffee mug, a special pen, a yummy meal, or an interesting book you are reading. Pick one of the photos of yourself and upload it to your profile. Post interesting facts that you learned from grand rounds or a study question. Share the latest data and studies on one of your core topics.

Finally, connect! Search for people in your field and search for people who inspire you. Follow them. Search for #hashtags (phrases without spaces preceded by the "#" sign which allows them to be searchable) for more interesting people to follow. Some examples are #medtwitter, #womeninmedicine, #tweetiatrician, and #meded. If you enjoy positivity, you can also search for #gratitude, #mindset, or #kindness. You can also follow hospital systems and specialty organizations.

Is following people all we have to do to make friends at the party? No! You can't just walk around and follow people. You have to also talk to them. Engage in the conversation by liking and replying to intriguing posts or questions. You can also share posts. On Twitter, sharing is also known as "retweeting." When you "quote retweet" on Twitter, you are sharing someone's post but also adding your own thoughts that you feel are kind of important. Don't do this too often, because it detracts from the original person's post. Let other people speak and show up on your timeline (list of your posts or shares). Be mindful to share or retweet content from a diverse crowd. Share the dance floor with others.

Now, how cool would it be if we could all party at the same time, instead of having broken up conversations? That's basically what a "Twitter chat" is. On a predetermined date and time, one account will post questions every 10 to 15 minutes for 1 hour. People will respond to those questions and comment on each other's posts. This is a great way to find and connect with people in real time. You can find chats by searching (e.g., "hospitalist chat") or by asking in a post (e.g., "Which chats should I follow on hospital medicine?") or by messaging someone with similar interests for recommendations.

Etiquette

The most important rule to remember when using social media as a healthcare professional is, of course, complying with the Health Insurance Portability and Accountability Act (HIPAA). A good test of whether or not a post complies with HIPAA is asking yourself if you would feel comfortable sharing this at a cocktail party where everyone is invited or on a crowded elevator. If you do share, avoid exposing patient identifiers by altering as many details as you can, such as the date of encounter, age, and physical and personality features.

Another question to determine if something is appropriate to share is to ask what purpose does this post/photo serve? For example, even if a patient allows a photo to be taken and no identifying features are exposed, consider if it truly adds a lot of educational value. Is this type of photo not available in a book or journal? And if not, consider publishing it instead of posting it. Let's also consider a celebratory post about a champagne tap or being right about diagnosing a rare cancer. What educational value does that add? While our achievements should be recognized, consider that it may also be the reason for a family's suffering. It is probably best to share these victories with your in-real-life circle. Lastly, be aware of your employer's social media usage guidelines. Many of these tips probably also align with company policies.

Here are two of my rhymes to finish off this section on how to behave on social media.

"Think twice, tweet nice." –Joannie Yeh MD

Be kind. Intentions are difficult to interpret without visual cues, sometimes without context. Assume good intent and move on. Add kind words if you have them. Still, people might attack. They are called trolls. They lose power when they are ignored. Don't feel like you need to write something back if you don't want to. It's okay to respond with silence. It's okay respond by blocking them. Save yourself from drama. Focus on where you can add value.

"Check the source before you endorse." –Joannie Yeh MD

There's a lot of information on the internet. Some of it looks very enticing and curious. Be careful what you share. Do the research. Read the full article before sharing it. As healthcare professionals, one of our purposes on social media is to increase public awareness of data and stories that help that data make sense to the lay public. Let's not confuse people by inadvertently sharing a click-baity article that may sound good but skews data to fit a sensationalized and dishonest narrative. Also, check a person's profile before you follow them or share their content.

Despite your best intentions, there will also be shady characters on social media that are relentlessly mean, persistently posting false information, or inappropriate. Feel free to utilize the block and report options for these accounts. Protect your time, because you have other projects to get to, such as the writing and speaking assignments (see next section).

Writing, Speaking and Beyond

The social media platforms can only help you do so much to network and connect with others. If you want to get a larger audience and reach or if you want to write longer posts about the topics you establish an expertise in, here are a few outlets to explore. You can guest post on someone's blog or start your own. This is a great way to just practice writing about your core topics and finding your style. You can submit articles to physician platforms like KevinMD and Doximity. You can also talk about your topics as a guest or host on a podcast.

To reach nonmedical audiences, consider working with your employer's communications manager to explore opportunities to be interviewed by local news channels, radio shows, and magazines. Another option is to submit a letter to the editor or op-ed to a newspaper to share your opinion about a recent article or event. Check individual newspaper websites for their submission guidelines. The Help A Reporter Out (HARO) website is another way to share your voice. It is an online tool that connects you to a reporter when they are looking for a quote from someone with your specific expertise.

Final Thoughts

Keep your engagement consistent and mind your boundaries. When you first start, make a schedule for when to post and interact, so you don't feel so lost trying to figure out who to talk to and which hashtags to use. Maybe just 10 minutes once a day. Remember, be patient. Just like how you usually don't become best friends with people you meet for the first time at a cocktail party, making friends and developing meaningful connections on social media is a gradual process. Over time, using the ACE purposes and profile suggestions, you will find your people and they will find you.

As you build and find your community, also be empowered to say no if you don't want to connect with someone or if you don't have time to answer private messages. Trolls on social media, incessant flow of the news, or events in your own life can make hanging out on social media not helpful or healthy for you. It's okay to take a break (as I take a 1-month break from Twitter while writing this chapter). Decide on your boundaries without apology.

Social media is an amazing cocktail party where you can be inspired by people from all over the world and have the chance to inspire others. I'll see you out there on the dance floor.

References

1. Eysenbach G. Can tweets predict citations? Metrics of social impact based on twitter and correlation with traditional metrics of scientific impact. J Med Internet Res. 2011;13(4):e123. https://www.jmir.org/2011/4/e123.
2. Jay WR, Jay M, Angelina W, Aase Lee A, Lanier William L, Timimi Farris K, Gerber Thomas C. Effect of promotion via social media on access of articles in an academic medical journal: a randomized controlled trial. Acad Med. 2019;94(10):1546–53.
3. https://www.kantarmedia.com/us/thinking-and-resources/blog/who-are-the-physicians-using-social-media.

Part VI

Maintaining Your Health

Having Perspective: Personal Health and Family Life

Jodi Brady-Olympia
and Robert P. Olympia

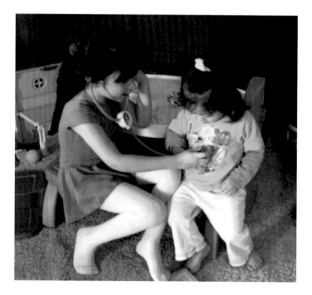

J. Brady-Olympia (✉)
Department of Pediatrics, Penn State Children's Hospital,
Hershey, PA, USA
e-mail: jbradyolympia@pennstatehealth.psu.edu

R. P. Olympia
Department of Emergency Medicine & Pediatrics, Penn State Hershey
Medical Center, Hershey, PA, USA
e-mail: rolympia@hmc.psu.edu

P. M. Garrett, K. Yoon-Flannery (eds.), *A Pediatrician's Path*,
https://doi.org/10.1007/978-3-030-75370-2_53

We became better pediatricians when our daughters were born. Questions of "why would you come to the ER for something so non-life threatening?" or "why are adolescent medicine physicians replacing primary care physicians?" now made sense after our children were born. Although we learned about the science of medicine in medical school (Penn State College of Medicine for Jodi and Jefferson Medical College for Robert) and residency (DuPont Hospital for Children for both of us), being parents has given us an even greater appreciation for the art of medicine. Our goals of being the Division Chief of Pediatric Emergency Medicine or Professor of Pediatrics within the Division of Adolescent Medicine were tempered with the realization that our children would take up most of our time and effort. And we didn't mind the "sacrifice" one bit.

Being the personal Uber for our children, devoting a significant portion of our salaries toward their education and futures, and spending time down at Walt Disney World (yes, we are a Disney Junkies family) suddenly replaced meetings at work, time spent obtaining grants, and traveling all over the country attending conferences and scientific assemblies. Our lives changed when we had our daughters, and we consciously decided to adjust with these changes.

Personal Health Is the Ultimate Form of Wellness

Your health is not just your past medical history, the medications you take, or your vital signs. Personal health is a conscious decision to choose wellness in every aspect of your life, not just your physical well-being, but also includes aspects of your emotional, spiritual, financial, social, and intellectual states. Achieving personal health is not just feeding your body but nourishing your mind and spirit. The importance of making time for self-care and personal health cannot be overemphasized. Factors associated with the prevention of burnout among pediatricians include focusing on personal health and having supportive physician colleagues, while factors associated with decreased overall satisfaction include inadequate sleep and working greater than 50 hours per week [1].

Balance Is the Key to Personal Health and Family Life

The key to personal health and family life is balance. As physicians, we are pulled in many different directions: work, family, personal interests, and community responsibilities. While your professional career often takes a significant portion of your time and effort, unless you have balance in your life outside of medicine, you won't achieve happiness or success in those areas of your life. Being in balance is about aligning what we do with what we value. Finding balance is being ourselves in the truest sense. It is discovering your passions in life, and prioritizing these passions in the structure of your day, week, month, and year. It is setting goals, both long term and short term. And if you are married and/or have children, fitting family life into this balancing act can be challenging, but rewarding in the end.

How Do You Attain Balance in Your Lives?

There are three steps to successfully attaining balance in your life:

1. *Develop a reflective practice:* Set aside time to reflect on a regular basis …each day, each week, or once a month. Select a routine that fits into your schedule, but make sure that this time of reflection is without distractions. Externalize these thoughts, either with paper and pen, laptop, or electronic device. Reinforce and extend your self-reflections with your significant other, your family, friends, and/or colleagues and mentors.

2. *Reflect on your life priorities:* As mentioned previously, the key to personal health is consciously choosing wellness, finding what your passions are, and balancing and prioritizing

these passions. Answering the following questions can help framework this reflection:

- What do you hold precious in your heart about your life?
- In what moments do you feel alive and well?
- What gives you satisfaction and fulfillment?
- Are your energies devoted to what holds meaning and worth for you?
- When you have lived your life and are reflecting back on it, how will you want it to look?

3. *Consider your life responsibilities:* Attaining personal health can't be that easy, can it? No matter what, there will always be obstacles to overcome on your road to personal health. Answering the following questions can help identify these obstacles:

- Is the time and effort you are currently investing in certain aspects of your life moving you toward goals that are important to you?
- If your life is balanced more in favor of your professional career, is the work meaningful to you?
- Are the financial securities and benefits allowing you to have meaning elsewhere in your life?
- Are there other tangible and intangible rewards?
- Are you sacrificing too much for future goals?
- Where is the right place for you to set the line between work investment and personal life?

Let's Spin the Balance of Life Wheel

The Balance of Life Wheel Assessment is a tool often used for coaching and personal development. The tool consists of eight categories formed around a wheel that are potentially important for attaining personal health and finding balance. Determining your present level of satisfaction for each category and then connecting the dots for each category identifies areas around the wheel that may create imbalance. These categories include the following:

– Career	– Leisure and recreation
– Family	– Money
– Friends	– Spirituality and personal growth
– Romance/significant other	– Fitness and health

Once you identify your current level of satisfaction (7 = completely satisfied to 1 = completely dissatisfied) for each category in the wheel, complete the following table:

Category	Current level of satisfaction (7–1)	Present time/ energy (%)	Importance in your life (0–100%)	Future time/ energy (%)	Anticipated obstacles
Career					
Family					
Friends					
Romance					
Leisure					
Money					
Spirituality					
Fitness/ health					
Total		= 100%		= 100%	

Setting Goals

Once you have identified and prioritized aspects of your life based on your current state of personal health and where you want to be, taking in account anticipated obstacles, it's time to set goals. Utilizing the SMART mnemonic, these goals should be specific, measurable, achievable, realistic, and timely [2]. Provide short-term and long-term visions. Write a personal statement. Publically announce your goals and ask for follow-up and reinforcement from family and friends.

Advice on Attaining Personal Health from Two Pediatric Parents

We don't claim to be the experts (our children slept in our bed many nights and both have technologic personal devices that they sometimes spend too much time on), but here are some suggestions based on 9 and 13 years of parental experience, and 20 years of married life:

> *Communication is key.* Seems logical and so easy, but fitting in time during the day to listen and express can be difficult when there are so many distractions. But it is a must. Perceived support from those around you, particularly family members, has been negatively correlated with emotional exhaustion and burnout, particularly among female physicians. This stresses the importance of devoting time to developing and maintaining social relationships [3]. One-on-one conversation, during a walk or after the children go to bed, is the key to finding balance in an unbalanced life. Sharing your goals and expectations, along with your frustrations and obstacles, with your significant other and/or children may lead to happiness and an "it's us against the world" approach to life.
>
> *Your family can't be happy unless you are happy.* Taking time for yourself in a busy world to reflect, relax, and rewind, apart from the family, is so important. For both Jodi and I, it's often when we work out or go for a run. Being happy and satisfied with your professional life reflects on your personal life, and vice versa. Continue to evaluate and prioritize aspects of your life, investing time and effort toward aspects that make you happy and cause little stress. Don't sweat the small stuff. Find personal time and space by creating an environment that enhances your comfort, concentration, and efficiency, protecting this environment from intrusions and avoiding interruptions.

Find out the passions of each member of your family and share these together (even if they don't interest you one bit). Making sacrifices is part of being a family. Going to see Sesame Street Live or visiting the American Girl Store in NYC wasn't always on our bucket lists, but the smiles on our children's faces made these experiences priceless. At the end of your life, you won't remember your total lifetime gross salary, the number of publications you've presented, or how many patient lives you've saved or impacted … we will remember those memories shared with family, friends, and our children.

Find a mentor. As important as it is to have a mentor in your professional career, it's equally important to have a role model to guide you in your personal life. A life coach, per se. Throughout our careers, we have encountered physicians who were not only successful in their professional lives but were amazing parents, community leaders, and friends. They were physicians that we strived to become and made the most impact in our lives.

Saying "no" is the hardest part. This is so important to maintaining personal health balance, but so difficult. We are wired to satisfy the needs of others, both professionally and personally. But as previously mentioned, our personal health is of utmost importance, and aligning our priorities and goals within the limited time structure of our lives should be maintained. While it is important to honor commitments and responsibilities at work, we also need to know when it is important to say "I'm sorry, but I can't make that meeting, my daughter has a basketball game." In the same way that we tell the parents of our patients that it is important to take time off from work to come to an important appointment, we need to follow that same advice in order to care for our own children.

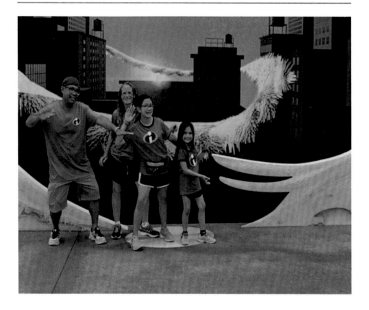

References

1. Starmer AJ, Frintner MP, Freed GL. Work-life balance, burnout, and satisfaction of early career pediatricians. Pediatrics. 2016;137(4):e20153183.
2. Doran GT. There's a S.M.A.R.T. way to write management's goals and objectives. Manag Rev. 1981;70(11):35–6.
3. Wang L, Wang H, Shao S, Jia G, Xiang J. Job burnout on subjective well-being among Chinese female doctors: the moderating role of perceived social support. Front Psychol. 2020;11:435.

Setting Boundaries

54

Parisa M. Garrett

Introduction

Although medical professionalism demands that physician-patient boundaries be set and observed, this topic is often overlooked during pediatric training [1]. Other specialties, particularly psychiatry, do a better job preparing residents for these challenges. Aside from outright unethical behavior, such as sexual relations or abuse, boundaries are often blurry, and navigation is left to the physician's discretion.

Regarding physician-patient boundaries, opinions vary widely. Some physicians believe that any discussion beyond the scope of medical care is off-limits. For example, those with stricter boundaries may feel that disclosing information about their personal life or providing services beyond the scope of routine medical care should be avoided at all costs. Others believe that sharing these details or facilitating solutions to systemic barriers enhances the patient-physician relationship and results in better compliance and more meaningful care [2]. Some institutions provide guidelines delineating boundaries; others do not [3].

P. M. Garrett (✉)
Philadelphia Department of Public Health, Ambulatory Health Services, Philadelphia, PA, USA
e-mail: parisa.garrett@phila.gov

Regardless, there are many ways that boundaries may be pushed during your relationship with a patient and their family, and it's important to be prepared for these circumstances when they arise. This chapter will discuss some frequently encountered situations in the physician-patient relationship, or in the case of pediatrics, the physician-patient-parent relationship.

Receiving Gifts

Patients or parents may bring you gifts, particularly around the holidays or after receiving help with an especially concerning health issue [4]. Some institutions follow a gift policy with explicit limitations, but often it is left to the physician to determine whether to accept a gift. Most commonly, the gift's significance is in the act of giving it, not in its monetary value. Acceptance of small gifts may strengthen your relationship with the patient and family, with little downside. Refusal of such a gift may even be offensive to the family or viewed as disrespectful in some cultures. Over the years I have received many cards and edible treats from families, usually around the holidays, which I have happily accepted and shared with my colleagues and staff. If a gift makes you feel uncomfortable, however, because of its value or character, or because it feels like there may be strings attached, it is important to set and maintain a boundary. You can do this by expressing your concern, making clear your intention not to accept, and presenting other options by suggesting they gift it elsewhere or make a donation in your name.

Touching

While sexual touching is obviously off-limits, is it okay to hug a patient or parent? Pediatrics is unique in that we may hold our infant and toddler patients to bring them to the exam table or while examining them. Many preschool-age patients hug us hello or goodbye, and for many of us, this is part of what drives our love for pediatrics. But how about older children? I sometimes will touch the arm of a tween or teenage patient while talking if I am expressing concern or want their full attention. I have hugged young adult patients as they go off to college or transition to adult care, but I always first ask "can I hug you?" I find that these encounters strengthen the physician-patient relationship and are noncontroversial, especially since the parent is usually present as well. I have also hugged patients' mothers (always after asking permission first) if they were moving away, or during times of grief. As a female physician, I have never hugged a patient's father, nor have I been in a situation where I had considered it or felt that it would be natural to do so. As you begin practicing on your own, you will have to decide what feels comfortable for you, taking into consideration both the setting and your relationship with the family.

Living in the Community Where You Work

Living in the community where you work adds an additional layer of complication, as a patient or parent may have access to your personal contact information through the school or community directory. For over 10 years, I lived in the community where I worked. Some of my kids' friends were my patients, and I was friends with some of my patients' parents. I fielded many questions at the pool, at school pickup, and at sporting events. Many times, the question simply was, "should my child be seen in your office for this?" Anything beyond that, like looking at a rash or abrasion, answering questions about development, or discussing specific symptoms, I would document as I would any on-call conversation.

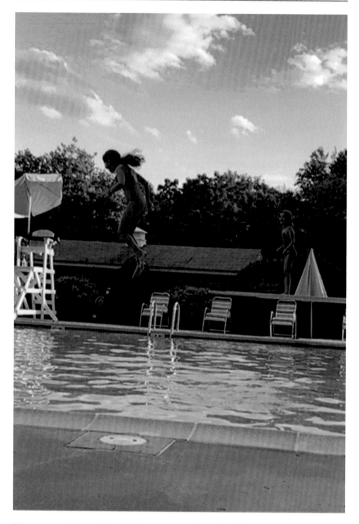

The community pool - one place you may be asked for medical advice

Likewise, if a parent calls you at home about a medical question, it should be handled the way an after-hours call from any patient is handled, with appropriate documentation. If the contact is initiated via personal email or social media, you can direct the parent or patient to contact the office through appropriate channels, or you can call them directly and document as you would any other patient call. During my 11 years of practice in my community, I was fortunate in that I was only contacted inappropriately once through social media and once through my child's class email list. Both times, I directed the parent to call our office for advice.

Helping a Patient Beyond the Scope of Medical Care

Once, about 12 years into my career, I called and paid for a car service to take my patient to the emergency room of the nearest children's hospital. The family had recently immigrated to the United States, was non-English speaking, and had neither the means to pay for a car service nor the knowledge to navigate public transportation to their destination. It was 4 pm on a Friday afternoon, and the child needed evaluation before the weekend. The car service was a $15 out-of-pocket expense for me and provided peace of mind that my patient was able to get to the hospital. This was a first for me, as I had never before given a patient a gift or offered to help financially. Although it was beyond the scope of traditional medical care, in those extenuating circumstances, for that small amount of money, it seemed like the right decision.

I haven't offered financial help to a patient again since that incident, but it does beg the question, "how does helping a patient beyond the scope of traditional medical care impact the relationship?" I have printed coupons for medications, called pharmacies to see which medications were available, and checked prices for the patient. I have recommended nanny agencies and daycares. Colleagues have helped patients find jobs and have written letters of recommendation. They have allowed patients to shadow them to build their resumes. When does helping a patient become crossing the line? You will have to decide for yourself, but going above and beyond must be done without expecting anything in return, and without the patient feeling like they are indebted to you.

Treatment Request by a Non-patient

If you are a clinical pediatrician, especially if you are doing primary care, you will be approached by friends, family, and acquaintances in the community for advice or treatment. This can be a sticky situation if the child is not your patient, or if the person seeking care is an adult. If asked to give advice to an adult, it is fair to answer that since you are a pediatrician, you may not be the best person to answer questions about adult medicine. Then you can advise them to call their own primary physician. For children who are not my patients, often I will give a vague answer of what I would consider if it were my patient and then advise them to discuss with their pediatrician. Even for my own children, I often seek advice from our pediatrician instead of treating them myself. Providing care to someone who is not your patient is risky, as you don't know their complete medical history. Additionally, there may be ethical issues associated with treating children of your family members or close friends. Treating an adult when you are a pediatrician adds even more liability. That being said, you have to decide for yourself where to draw the line. Refilling your mother's thyroid medication when she can't reach her own physician is very different from treating your adult neighbor for pneumonia. While these scenarios are perhaps two ends of the spectrum, there are countless variations in between that you will have to navigate using your best judgment.

As described, these are just a few ways in which your professional boundaries may be pushed, and there are many other situations you may encounter. Unless your institution has specific guidelines, establishing and sticking to boundaries are mostly up to you as the physician. A good rule of thumb is that if a situation makes you uncomfortable, it should be examined more closely and given thoughtful consideration before moving forward. Maintaining professionalism is essential to your success as a physician, but showing your human side also helps build the physician-family relationship.

References

1. Lewis J, Allan S. Physician-patient boundaries: professionalism training using video vignettes. MedEdPORTAL. 2016;12:10412. https://www.ncbi.nlm.nih.gov/pmc/articles/PMC6464555/.
2. Kaonga N. Professional boundaries and meaningful care. AMA J Ethics. 2015;17(5):416–8. https://journalofethics.ama-assn.org/article/professional-boundaries-and-meaningful-care/2015-05.
3. Petersen A. The new boundaries between doctors and patients. The Wall Street Journal website. December 7, 2015. Accessed 2 Jan 2021. https://www.wsj.com/articles/the-new-boundaries-between-doctors-and-patients-1449508150.
4. Committee on Bioethics. American Academy of Pediatrics Policy Statement—Pediatrician-Family-Patient Relationships: Managing the Boundaries. 2009. https://pediatrics.aappublications.org/content/pediatrics/124/6/1685.full.pdf. Accessed 2 Jan 2021.

Stress Management

55

Kahyun Yoon-Flannery

As a breast surgeon with four young kids all under the age of 10, I have personally dealt a lot with the concept of *stress*. My work life consists of patients who either are diagnosed with breast cancer or those who are there to rule out the diagnosis of breast cancer. Everyday I experience conversations full of anger, despair, denial, and hope, counseling patients and their loved ones through one of the most difficult times in their lives. Then I come home to a gaggle of screaming kids who are ready to pounce and ask for food because they apparently have been starving all day, and a husband.

After being newly diagnosed with hypertension, enough to be placed on a medication, I was recommended to *slow down*. This was a term that was unfamiliar to me. The level of defeat I felt however, to have to accept a medication regimen to bring down my elevated blood pressure, was extraordinary. I was born to be a surgeon. We surgeons are hammers. The concept of *needing* something on a daily basis made me realize that I had to change how I lived my life. I got to work, working to figure out strategies to manage my day-to-day stress, both at work and at home with my crazy family. I first sat down with my husband. I admitted that I needed help and that I would like to try a session or two of yoga.

K. Yoon-Flannery (✉)
Janet Knowles Breast Cancer Center, MD Anderson Cancer Center at Cooper, Camden, NJ, USA
e-mail: yoon-flannery-kay@cooperhealth.edu

I expected him to balk at this "ploy" to get out of the house and away from the chaos with the kids, but he surprised me. He said that he wanted me to take this time to focus on my wellness.

I formed a regimen consisting of a daily meditation routine along with yoga sessions, both restorative and rigorous, two to three times a week in person, supplemented by additional sessions using an app at home. My morning yoga session started at 5:30 in the morning, which made me feel like I was back in residency. But it felt invigorating to just be able to say that I was doing this for myself. I downloaded an app called Headspace and listened to the meditation sessions during my daily commute. I sat down to reevaluate my life in general, particularly with regard to stress from work. And I made a decision to accept an incredible job offer from a different institution. My blood pressure finally went down to normal. The new routine felt *normal*, after about a month.

Then the COVID-19 pandemic hit.

If you search "stress management" in Google, 797,000 results appear, including videos, self-help books, as well as numerous sites endorsed by medical societies. Stress management, according to the Mayo Clinic, consists of managing stress from physical and psychological standpoints.

Since the outbreak of COVID-19 pandemic, fortunately, there has been an outpouring of resources for stress management, particularly for healthcare workers. As I have been able to reassess my day-to-day life comprehensively, I am able to share the following guidelines for stress management, both in the workplace and in your personal life.

On the Job

1. *Do a self-evaluation.* If you have never sat down to figure out what is and isn't going well in your job, take a moment to do it now. And if you have done that, make a note to do this on a recurring basis. What are your goals; are they being achieved? If they are not, what are the barriers?
2. *Make a list of priorities and put them in the order of importance.* Make a timeline for each item and recategorize based on the timeline between goals for now vs. later.

3. *Find what your strengths and weaknesses are.* Are you having trouble closing charts on a daily basis? Not meeting deadlines for research? After identifying the issues on hand, write down your proposed solutions.

4. *Schedule breaks for lunch.* This is important. Even if you are catching up on labs or callbacks, we all need catch-up time between patients.

5. *Learn to say no.* Maintain a strict schedule protecting your off-work time. Saying no is the hardest thing we can do, but we must from time to time to maintain our sanity.

6. *Look around for other opportunities.* A wise friend said to me once that the grass is not greener on the other side; it's just that the brown patches are in different spots. Sometimes it takes looking elsewhere to stay happy where you are, or it may convince you to leave. It is always good to know your worth in your work community, particularly if you have issues in your current job that are beyond repair.

Off the Job

1. *Maximize time management* – If you have a family, maximize your spending time with them. The chores, cooking and other household work, may need to wait.

2. *Hire help.* Your time is valuable – Whether at work or at home. It is worth hiring someone to help unload household work so you can enjoy your time with family. The best thing I ever did was to hire help for cleaning. We will obviously have to keep things tidied up, but I no longer worry about spending time cleaning my toilets. I can now spend it yelling at my kids during "family time."

3. *Plan for vacations.* We all need to get away from it all – And we need something to look forward to. With the pandemic, all of our vacation plans for the foreseeable future obviously changed. It also showed us that we should never take things for granted. Plan for that vacation you always wanted.

4. *Schedule your "me" time.* We as physicians tend to prioritize everything else except us. Our patients, practice, and our family members. But we also need to focus on ourselves, no matter how little time we can preserve for that. Whether it is a massage on a

monthly basis, to a few minutes on a Sunday morning before everyone wakes up to read your journals, to going running every morning, carve out time only for yourself and do not feel guilty.

Stress management has several components I personally have found. Self-evaluation, or reevaluation of your current situation, is the first step. What is your day-to-day activity like? What are the major stressors in your life currently? And what can you change about those stressors and what remain an unchangeable component of your life? We all have probably spent countless hours and years fighting against the current, trying to change what is an immovable object. For years, I struggled at work trying to improve components of my own program. What could I contribute to change the process for my patients? What components in our radiological services need to be improved? What support services need to be provided from our administration? Then one day I sat down and realized, these are things I cannot personally change. So what could I change in this circumstance? I changed jobs.

Now telling someone to change one's job may seem to be a drastic move. But I hope you get the point in that we all have to slow down and reevaluate our current situation. Continuing to run into a wall is not going to bring a good outcome no matter what type of extreme stress management you can employ yourself. But figuring out which column of "changeability" a certain situation belongs to can certainly move the compass along.

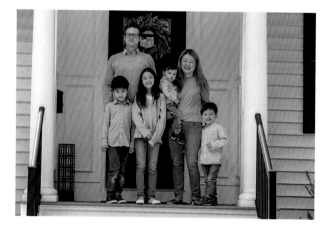

1. One of the best things about the pandemic – Spending time
   with family

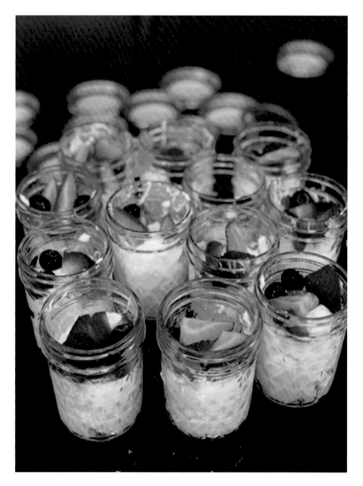

2. Second best thing about the pandemic – Experimenting with cooking

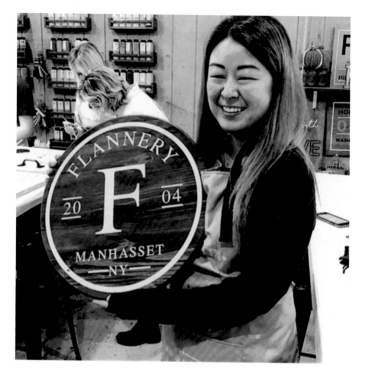

3. Fostering creativity can lead to stress management in the most positive way

Developing Interests Outside of Medicine and Avoiding Burnout

56

Sarah Kramer

So now you've been working in your practice for 5 or 10 years. You have endless charting and phone calls to catch up on, and you're working 2 weekend days a month. Oh, and you take call too. And you're being pushed all the time to see more patients. How can you avoid burning out? Is it possible? Many studies have shown high levels of physician burnout in all fields. According to the Medscape National Physician Burnout & Suicide Report 2020 (with over 15,000 responses), 41% of pediatricians report feeling burned out, and 49% of all physicians would take a pay cut to have more free time. The percentages are similar across all types of practices. 300–400 physicians commit suicide every year, and about 22% have had thoughts of suicide.

The first thing to realize is that it's rarely the patients, or even their parents, that cause the burnout. Most doctors who feel burned out state that they still like patient care. It's everything else that piles up – consult notes, labs, charting, phone calls, and forms. Plus, you have a life outside of the office – partners, children, parents, and friends all want and need some of your time as well.

There are things you can do to help yourself not feel burnt out. First of all, and most importantly, make sure you do not lose yourself. Do you sing? Go find a choir. Do you run? Get out there and go. Even though it may not feel like there are enough hours in the

S. Kramer (✉)
Watchung Pediatrics, Warren, NJ, USA
e-mail: skramer@watchungpediatrics.com

day, it doesn't take a lot of time to give yourself a little lift. It may not be as much or as often as you want, but you can't help your patients if you're not feeling yourself. When you started medical school, you didn't sign away your entire life and personality. Try to keep yourself fulfilled.

Which brings me to your family. The one you live with.

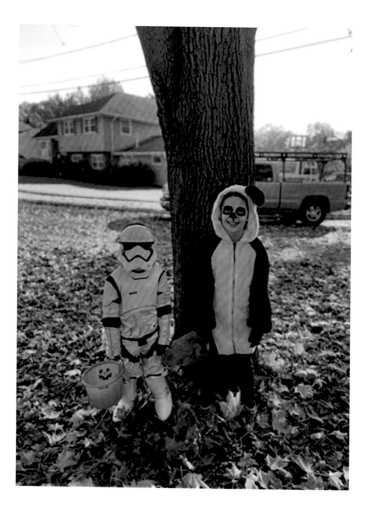

Anyone who tells you that it's possible to perfectly balance life and work is hiding something from you. No one can be a perfect parent, doctor, and partner all at the same time. The key is trying to make sure you keep work at work and home at home. This is of course easier said than done. The most important thing at work is *prioritizing*. If a patient has that much of an emergency that they want to reach you outside of hours, well, they don't need you, they need an emergency room. If you've arranged ahead of time to check in with a patient at night or on the weekends, by all means do so. You don't have to know about every refill requested or nonurgent call while you are gone. Reading most consult notes can wait. Some labs and phone calls cannot. As much as you can, do NOT bring work home.

On the other hand, when you're at work, you need to be able to push aside home concerns and focus on your patients. This is also easier said than done, and sometimes it's not possible. There are, of course, life events that are very consuming. Know when to speak up and say that you need help, whether it be some days off or lightening your schedule. You cannot be your best doctor self when you or a family member is ill. Knowing your limits in terms of your physical and mental health is very important.

Take your vacation!!! Vacation means you are not checking emails, and not logging into your electronic medical record. Part of being in a group practice (which most physicians are) means that you always have someone there who can cover for you.

Pediatrics provides many opportunities for part-time work. However, once you have your schedules, you usually have little to no flexibility to change a day at the last minute. When my daughter was in preschool, I found out I was going to be the only mom not at the Mother's Day celebration. I cried, which made the teacher cry. They gave us 3 weeks' notice, which is plenty for most professions, but not medicine. I was lucky enough to be able to move a few patients into my lunch hour, which cleared up the time I needed to go. These things are important to you as a parent and to your child. Do your best. You may not have time to be a room parent, but you might be able to help with a holiday celebration. Also, know that your kids will be proud of what you do for a living! My kids tell their friends that their mommy helps sick kids. When you put it like that, how much better does it get?

In terms of office paperwork, we've found ways to ease the burden in my practice. We have scribes who type during our visits, give the specialist lists to the patients, and fill in the school notes. They also read and summarize the consult notes, so all we have to do is read the summary and not spend time entering it into the EMR. The EMR also provides a lot of checkboxes and drop-down menus, which saves time. We've also gone to one-on-one nursing, which has been very helpful to streamline the day as well.

ALWAYS remember that you're part of a team, including your nurses and staff! I'm lucky to work at a practice where most of us really are friends. We are a support system for each other. It's so important to be able to lean on other people when you need to.

I was recently reminded of another way to help with burnout. I participate in a yearly program that gives rising juniors and seniors in college the opportunity to shadow a doctor in a different specialty every day for a month. This year, amidst the COVID-19 pandemic, things were obviously different. Instead of the students coming into the office, I gave a zoom session about pediatrics. Showing others what you do can be a great source of renewal. It reminds you of the good things, and why you went into medicine in the first place. So if there's an opportunity to teach, to have a shadow, or to speak about your career, take it. It really can remind you why you did this in the first place.

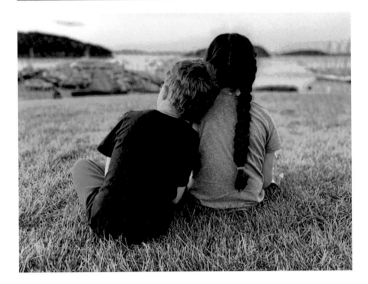

Index